COMPLETE BODYWEIGHT TRAINING COLLECTION FOR BEGINNERS AND SENIORS

7x Your Strength Gains + Shredded Secrets

The Muscle Building and Bodybuilding Diet Boxset Even If You Are a Man or Woman Over 50

REX BONDS

TABLE OF CONTENTS

PART 2 – FUNDAMENTAL EXERCISES

SHREDDED SECRETS: BUILD MUSCLE, BURN FAT.. 153

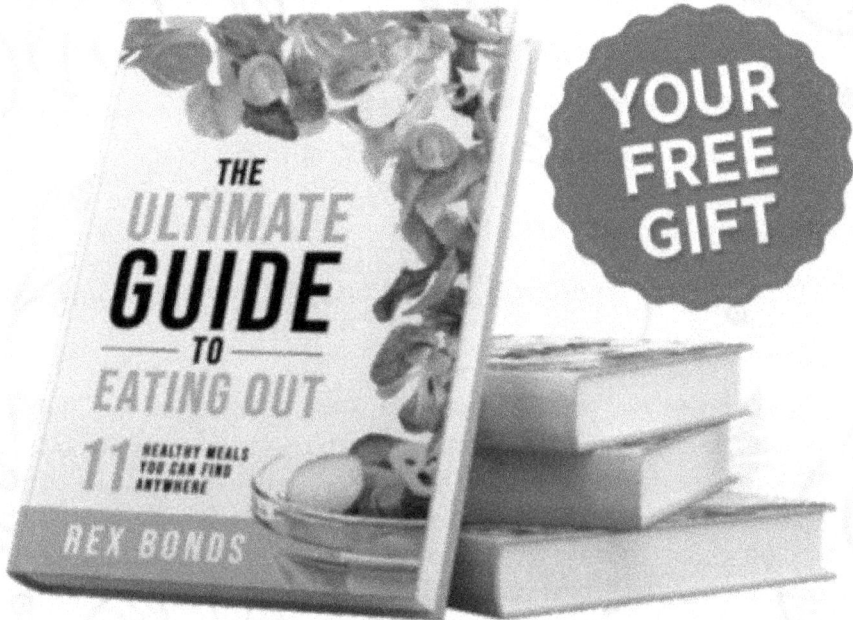

THE
ULTIMATE
GUIDE
TO
EATING OUT

11 HEALTHY MEALS
YOU CAN FIND
ANYWHERE

REX BONDS

YOUR FREE GIFT

Before we get started, I'd like to offer you this free gift. It's my way of saying thank you for spending time with me in this book. Your gift is a Special Report titled, *"The Ultimate Guide To Eating Out: 11 Healthy Meals You Can Find Anywhere."* It's an easy-to-use guide that pulls together a ton of analysis I've previously only shared with clients. I think you're going to love it. This guide is a collection of 11 Healthy Meals you can find anywhere that will give you the system, tools, info, and mindset you need on the path to achieving your fitness dreams. This guide will teach you where to find clean, nutrition-packed meals to build lean muscle, burn fat and bump up your confidence in every situation no matter where you are.

**Scan Me
To Claim Your Free Gift!**

In this guide you'll learn:

- ✓ Where to find the 11 healthiest meals when you're eating out
- ✓ A rock-solid meal plan for any time of day & every location
- ✓ The exact script for which menu items to order
- ✓ Nutritional information for each dish at your fingertips

Plus as a Bonus!

- ✓ A Nutrition and fitness Journal to stay on track daily to your fitness dreams!

I'm willing to bet you'll find at least a few ideas, tools and meals covered in that guide that will surprise and help you. This guide will set you up for success and is a proven system when eating out. With this guide you will be armed with the info & focus you need. You will be giving your body nutritious fuel and enjoy eating out. With downloading this guide, you're taking a solid step on the path to your fitness success.

How can you obtain a copy of *The Ultimate Guide To Eating Out: 11 Healthy Meals You Can Find Anywhere?* It's simple. Visit RexBondsBooks.com and sign up for my email list (or simply click the link above). You'll receive immediate access to the Report in PDF format. You can read it online, download it or print it out. You will also get a Free Fitness Journal and Planner for signing up for my email list as well. Everything you need to get started and stay on your fitness journey is included in **signing up for my email list.**

Being on my email list also means you'll be the first to know when I release a new health and fitness book. I plan to release my books at a steep discount (or even free) for the first 24 hours. By signing up for my email list you'll get an early notification.

If you don't want to join my list, that's completely fine. This just means I need to earn your trust. With this in mind, I think you are going to love the information I've included in the ultimate guide. More specifically, I think you're going to love what it can do for your life.

Without further ado, let's jump into this book.

Join the Rex Bonds Fitness Community

Looking to build your specific fitness habits and goals? If so, then check out the Rex Bonds Fitness community: Rex Bonds Fitness Group

This is an amazing group full of like-minded individuals who focus on getting results with their lives. Here you can discover simple strategies, build powerful habits, find accountability partners and ask questions about your struggles. If you want to "level up" in your fitness journey, then this is the place to be.

**Just scan the QR code below
to join the Rex Bonds Fitness Community.**

7X YOUR STRENGTH GAINS EVEN IF YOU'RE A MAN, WOMEN OR CLUELESS BEGINNER OVER 50

Bodyweight Training Exercises and Workouts A.K.A. Calisthenics

REX BONDS

INTRODUCTION

Strength, muscles, stamina. Who doesn't want all three of them? While it would be great to have each in abundance, the fact is that the human body is designed to be great at either strength or stamina. Having said that, this doesn't mean your stamina needs to be terrible in order to maximize muscle. It is perfectly possible to have levels of strength and stamina that together ensure a healthy and happy life.

Unfortunately, attaining even a fraction of both of these things seems impossible for a lot of people. The fitness industry doesn't make things any easier. There are seemingly endless fitness programs and workouts, all of which have fancy names, along with a list of supplements that promise to make you healthier than ever. Health itself is something that changes depending on who you're listening to.

The muscle building websites tell you to build as much strength as possible and train to exhaustion. The specialized program websites tell you that following their principles is the best, and then there's the MMA crowd that tells you to ditch the weight and start punching things. All of this can be aggravating to the extreme.

An additional concern for you, given that you've picked up this book, is age. If you're beyond 50, I hate to break it to you, but society now considers you old. Although whatever society might say, the fact is that your body is not what it used to be. When you were younger, you could get away with taking a few shortcuts with regard to your fitness and diet and still expect to function well.

These days though, slight deviations from what your body is regularly used to can potentially cause significant harm. Training for someone of your age is as much about preservation as it is about strength and stamina building. By preservation, I'm talking about your joints, tendons, and ligaments. In your younger days, you could get away with not knowing what these things were, but this is not the case now.

There are a lot of myths surrounding the muscle and strength building process for older people. One popular myth is that you cannot put on any muscle beyond the age of 30 and that you're better off running on a treadmill once past this age. Another myth is that the best workout for someone of your age is to simply walk briskly and to stay away from weights altogether since these might damage your joints.

When taken all together, it's no wonder that people over 50 are intimidated at the thought of getting fit. After all, if there are so many things to figure out and so many things to be careful of, is it even possible to get fit?

I'm here to tell you that yes, it absolutely is. What's more critical is that your life depends on it.

Fitness and Age

Let's face it: You're not getting any younger. I'm not trying to put you down but just highlighting that it is more important than ever for you to get serious about your fitness. I'm not saying you need to turn into Superman or Wonder Woman, but you should be able to climb a staircase without sounding like a banshee by the end of it.

The fact is that you're going to receive just one body in your lifetime. It is also a fact that it is going to start creaking as you get older. No matter how hard you try to avoid it, age is going to get you one day. The best thing you can do is to make this process as enjoyable as possible.

This means being able to play with your grandkids without clutching your back. This means being able to take care of yourself on family vacations without your loved ones having to research every doctor and medical facility in the area. It means giving your loved ones the least amount of headaches and not having to worry about your health all the time.

Health and exercise are priorities and responsibilities. I understand it is intimidating to begin, but this is precisely why I'm here. By the end of this book, you're going to gain deep knowledge on how to build your strength best and also how to design your own fitness program. You will be able to work on your fitness wherever you are, without having to worry about signing up for a gym membership or any other fancy workout course.

The question at this point is: why should you listen to me?

Trainer and Guide

I could list all of the accolades I've won over the years as a bodybuilder and a personal trainer. I could list all the testimonials from hundreds of my satisfied clients. Instead, I'll just say this: I've helped tons of clients who are over the age of 50, and I get it. As someone who's been in the fitness industry all my life, both as a customer and as someone who's sold his services to clients, I deeply understand how tough it is for someone to get started at an older age. The fact is that a lot of marketing that is prevalent in the industry is geared towards making you feel bad about yourself.

This sort of guilt-tripping and shaming is far worse when someone starts off late in life. The truth is that it is never too late to begin exercising correctly. Over my many years of experience, I've learned one unassailable fact: your body is your biggest asset when it comes to getting fit.

That might sound like a strange statement to make. Isn't fitness supposed to aid the body? How does the body aid fitness? The answer is bodyweight training. I've sustained and recovered from many weight lifting related injuries over the years, and those alone would be enough to make a great case.

I don't mean to say that weightlifting is bad or worse. It's just that for someone in your position, whether you're too busy to work out or whether you're just getting started and have no clue about how to train well, the fact is that bodyweight training is as close to risk-free as training can get, as well as being the most repeatable form of exercise.

Life gets in the way regularly, and it can be tough to set aside times during the day when you can go to the gym or go out for a run or a swim. By relying on bodyweight training routines, you can workout literally anywhere in the world. All you need to do is to find a place where you can stretch out your body a little bit. How easy is that?

I've been following the routine outlined in this book myself and have been prescribing it for my clients who are over the age of 50. In my case, I prevented a ton of common injuries most people have attained throughout their fitness journey. Bodyweight training isn't going to cause muscle loss or strength reduction as well. If anything, you'll be able to maintain your levels a lot better and also increase them.

You will learn actionable steps to take to your goals through this bodyweight training program, and you can now workout anywhere in the world, including right in your own living room. You will be working out with a lot less stress on your joints because it allows you to have a lot of more natural range of motions. Pains and kinks in your knees, elbows, and shoulders will fade away over the next year, and by practicing perfect form, you will have no injuries since starting the program. Your knees and ankles won't crack in the morning when you walk around the house, and you will be more limber and supple than you have ever been. All of your chronic pain will simply be gone. You're going to look lean and fit, but most importantly, you're going to truly feel lean and fit.

Benefits

All of my clients report higher levels of strength than before starting these routines. They're able to carry objects that were once too heavy for them and are not worried about sustaining joint injuries anymore. Not only are their strength levels up, but their stamina and endurance have also increased as well. Clients have been commenting on the increased muscle mass in their chest, back, and shoulders.

Some of my clients who've been lifting weights for years and have now switched to this routine are seeing even bigger benefits to their body and strength. The best part is the complete lack of injury to their ankles, wrists, and shoulders. All of these results could be yours. However, it requires you to understand one simple thing.

You need to act. The best time to have gotten started with this routine was 20 years ago. The second best time is right now. You've taken the first right step by purchasing this book. As you read through it, remember that every step in here is meant to be implemented, not read about, and then forgotten.

My promise to you is that once you begin implementing this routine, you'll have a body that doesn't just look strong but is strong and fit. All you need to do is act. After all, you owe it to yourself and your loved ones.

So without further ado, let's dive into the fundamentals of bodyweight training.

PART 1

SETTING THE FOUNDATIONS

CHAPTER 1:

THE CORE PRINCIPLES OF EVERYTHING YOU NEED TO KNOW ABOUT BODYWEIGHT STRENGTH TRAINING

So why is bodyweight training so effective? More importantly, if it is effective, why does weight training hog all the limelight and why do a lot of people think that it is superior to bodyweight training? This chapter is going to give you a few foundational principles you should keep in mind when you begin to exercise.

Most importantly, it is going to show you that you don't need fancy equipment or a gym to be able to get strong, lose fat, and build your stamina.

Why Bodyweight Training?

The word "training" most likely conjures images of a sweaty gym with people huddled over machines and dumbells moving to and fro. There's no doubt that training with weights is effective. I mean, I am a heavy weightlifter myself! However, to think that it is the only worthwhile form of training is a mistake.

Weightlifting has its positives, but one of the biggest negatives to do with it is the prevalence of injuries. In order to progress, you need to keep increasing the weight you lift. There eventually comes a point where you'll be close to your maximum strength limit, and with the intention of completing your exercise set, you'll end up injuring yourself since your body will simply fail.

Injuries sustained from weightlifting can be life-altering, especially if they involve your joints or back. Aside from injuries, it's no secret that these types of exercises place a massive load on your joints ("Most Common Weightlifting Injuries and 5 Tips to Avoid Them", 2019). You will also need tons of equipment to weight train correctly.

The Advantages of Bodyweight Training

This is where bodyweight training is far superior to weight lifting. All you need is your body. You don't need any equipment or accessories of any kind. The reason most people find bodyweight training ineffective is that they perform the exercises incorrectly.

For example, one of the most common bodyweight exercises is the pushup. It's pretty simple. Lie flat on your stomach and push yourself up off the ground. You'd be surprised at how many people fail to perform this exercise correctly and end up sustaining injuries to their shoulders and wrists.

It is possible to sustain injuries from any movement that is performed incorrectly. The form is what determines the likelihood of injury, not the type of exercise. The critical point is that the injuries you can potentially sustain when training with just your bodyweight will be far less severe than the ones you sustain from weight lifting. This is because your body is not being pushed past its limit to much.

Recovery and energy levels after a workout are higher on average with these types of exercises. You don't need to buy medicine balls or sign up for yoga classes to preserve flexibility unless you want to. Your body will be working within safe limits while pushing itself to grow stronger at the same time. Let's look at some of the benefits of bodyweight training in more detail.

You Don't Need a Gym or Accessories

This one is self-explanatory. You don't need special equipment for a pushup. Some exercises do need accessories, but even these are so easily obtained that it's laughable to think of them as accessories. For example, you need a bar of some kind to perform a pullup. This can be a particular accessory you purchase, or it can be a monkey bar you find on a playground or beach.

It can be a wooden or metal beam in your home or garage. It can be a tree branch. What I mean is that you're not going to have to spend too much time figuring out how to perform the exercise, but I still highly recommend buying an actual pull up bar for your home.

Optimum Power to Weight Ratio

Here's how progress in weightlifting occurs. You lift a certain amount of weight today and tomorrow (or some preset time limit later), you lift the weight that is one degree higher than it. The idea is that your muscles are continually being challenged and have to grow in order to make progress.

This works for the most part, but the problem is that your body isn't a machine. It has days when it isn't at its best. It has days when it needs ample rest. Forcing an arbitrary weight number on it externally will lead to injuries. Training this way also assumes that everyone's body responds the same way to training routines.

This is simply untrue since everyone's body is different. By training with your body weight, you're allowing your body the room to adjust and modulate how much energy it can devote to that particular exercise without overexerting itself. This prevents a lot of injuries that are commonplace when weight lifting.

Greater Flexibility and Balance

Thanks to your body having more room to work with (in terms of being able to better adjust to the weight it needs to push), it develops more agility and flexibility. The communication between the different parts of your body becomes better, and you'll find that you'll utilize your muscles far more efficiently.

For example, once you begin performing pushups, you'll notice your core becomes stronger, even though you're not directly exercising it. This will impact the way you walk, and you'll find yourself standing up straighter because your core is now more actively supporting you.

Weight training involves a lot of isolation exercises. You can train your biceps to look as good and robust as they can be, but when you lift something off the floor, you're using your legs, glutes, back, shoulder, core, and your biceps. If these muscles aren't used to talking to one another, the amount of weight you can lift in real life will not be equivalent to the weight you lift in the gym.

Bodyweight training simply avoids all of these issues by never having to isolate anything in the first place. Your sense of balance and flexibility will remain what they were before you began training and will even increase.

Clear Targets

Given that your body will be able to adjust far better to your training methods, you'll be able to set and hit your training targets better. A common occurrence in weight training regimes is stalling. This refers to when the trainee cannot lift beyond a certain amount of weight after a while.

Stalling occurs due to fatigue building up over time and the body reaching a level beyond which it cannot move forward without significant rest. Most trainees have no idea how to handle stalls, and it takes a bit of experience to move past one. There is no risk of stalling with bodyweight training since you're always within your body's limits.

In effect, it sets the rate of progress and the tone of your training. Thus, your goals are a lot clearer, and you're never in any doubt as to which level to aim for.

Variations

Our bodies are incredibly versatile and can adapt to a lot of situations. Once you begin training, you'll realize that your body will adjust and get used to that movement. As a result, progress occurs in shorter bursts, and you'll take longer to see the same level of gains as you previously experienced.

When this happens with weight training, you'll need to figure out different exercises to perform, which means learning new movements. With bodyweight training, adjustments are far easier to make. Sticking with the pushup, if you find your body adjusting to it, lift one of your legs off the floor the next time you do it.

Even better, place your legs on an elevation and push up from a decline. You can do the Rocky Balboa pushup where you pushup with one arm, explode at the top and come down on the other and repeat the action. You can bring your arms closer to your body or push wider. Lift both your legs off the ground etc etc. There is almost no end to the number of variations you can deploy when training like this. All of this enables you to keep surprising your body, and you'll make more constant and consistent progress.

Tailormade

Bodyweight training is an immensely flexible and versatile training method. Through such routines, you'll be able to work towards multiple goals at the same time since it helps develop your strength, endurance, and agility (Why bodyweight training, 2019). Furthermore, if you're looking at taking up a new sport, bodyweight training has a number of benefits for you since it will provide a strong foundation for any other form of activity.

The Most Common Training Mistakes - And How to Avoid Them

One of the reasons most exercise regimes fail is due to the fact that people commit some highly avoidable errors. A lot of these apply equally to bodyweight training routines. With this in mind, let's look at some of the mistakes that you should avoid.

Training Beyond Capacity

This mistake is almost impossible to commit when training with your body weight, but it still occurs. The most common way is when the trainee decides to get creative with their training and sticks an additional dumbbell or weight plate onto the exercise, and all of a sudden, the body is being pushed beyond its capacity.

Exercising Till Failure

Unlike the previous mistake, this one is eminently possible when training with just your bodyweight. This occurs mostly due to the stereotype that surrounds training hard. Common motivational sayings such as 'go hard or go home' and so on get people to think that unless they're puking their guts out, they haven't really trained.

The truth is that the ideal strength level you want to hit is around 90% of your maximum capacity. This means that you should stop performing the exercise when you feel that you'll tap out within a couple more repetitions of it. Admittedly, this is a feel based metric that will be difficult to figure out at first.

However, over time you'll get to know your body better and will avoid this mistake.

Lack of a Plan

How often have you seen people get dressed up in their fancy workout gear upon reaching the gym, and all they do is randomly train at various things before packing up to go home at the slightest hint of sweat? The fact is that you need to plan your training in the gym much before you decide to step into it.

This means having a clear and precise workout plan that lists how many repetitions or the interval for which you will perform an exercise. Not only does this planning need to be done for a daily session but also across sessions. How will you make sure you'll keep pushing yourself to the ideal limit?

This is where a workout routine helps immensely. It doesn't have to be fancy, but you need a basic plan in place. Anything else, and you'll end up looking clueless.

Too Many Reps

Rep is short for repetition, and high rep exercises are one of the most common mistakes that beginners make. It isn't just beginners, even people who have been training unsuccessfully for a while, end up committing this error. The reason this error occurs is that most people don't understand that training methods depend on goals.

To be honest, the weightlifting world is more susceptible to this than the bodyweight trainers. What usually happens is that a beginner goes to the gym and sees the hulk in the corner, lifting tiny weights for a large number of reps. The reason the hulk trains this way is because he already has a high level of strength, and these low weight/high rep routines give him a good pump.

A beginner is not going to see any benefit from these routines since they have no muscle to pump in the first place. They need to be working on building their strength before worrying about how they'll look. When performing bodyweight exercises, you want to concentrate on pushing your strength forward as much as possible instead of trying to perform an inordinately large number of reps for an exercise.

Ignoring Illness or Injury

One of the most perverse results that motivational speeches and quotes create is to get sick people to go workout instead of staying at home and getting better. Trying to train when sick is a bit like trying to run with one leg incapacitated. You're just not going to do it very well.

Even worse, training and exercise place stress on the body, and when sick, stress is the last thing you need. So be kind to yourself and lay off for a while. Injury is a tricky thing for most beginners because they cannot distinguish between soreness and injury.

Soreness is the result of a lack of blood flow through a particular area, whereas injury is the result of tissue damage. The former feels uncomfortable all the time but disappears once you perform the same movement that caused it, thereby forcing blood to flow through the muscle again. An injury will be accompanied by a sharp pain at all times or a pain when you try to perform the movement that caused it. You will also feel weakness in that area when you move it.

Learning to identify the difference between soreness and injury takes time. The key is to minimize the potential for injury before you learn the difference.

Inadequate Rest

No matter the routine you choose to follow, you need adequate amounts of rest. This is usually allowing a rest period of 24 hours between your workouts. As you become more experienced, you can shorten this since you'll know your body better. However, in the beginning, it's best to train on alternate days, especially when you're looking to build strength.

Rest periods are extremely important because true progress occurs when you rest, not when you train. It is during the resting period that your body repairs itself and breaks down existing muscle fibers to build bigger, stronger ones. This is where strength is built. So never underestimate your rest periods and always prioritize them.

Lack of a Warm-Up

Have you ever tried starting a car in the dead of winter? Or have you ever tried accelerating it to top speed immediately after you start the engine? If your car happens to be brand new, it won't need much of a warm-up period, but it is unlikely that the engine will be able to hit peak performance immediately. An old car might just die on you if you try to do this.

Your body is much the same. I'm not saying you're going to drop dead from a lack of warmups, by the way. What I mean is that you need to take the time to get the blood flowing to various parts of your body before pushing it close to its limit. This is common sense, but most people who train don't follow this simple rule.

They jump in and immediately try to lift the weight they're supposed to lift during that session. This is the easiest way to injure yourself. You might have gotten away with it when you were younger, but trying to do this at your current age is a terrible idea.

Ignoring Nutrition

When you exercise, you burn calories. Your body is placed under stress, and to recover, it needs food (fuel). Not eating well and eating inadequate amounts of food is one of the most significant mistakes trainees make. To be honest, this mistake usually occurs due to a lack of planning.

Plan your meals ahead of time, so you're not going to come home to an empty kitchen or fridge after your workout. Grabbing some fast food after your workout might be fine once or twice, but you don't want to make a habit of this. Remember that as you grow older, you're going to need to pay more attention to the micronutrients in your food, such as the vitamins and minerals.

Junk food is full of processed chemicals that give you a short term sugar rush but nothing in terms of nutrition. So plan your meals and quantities ahead of time and make sure you don't go hungry and undo all your progress.

Improper Macros

Macros refer to macronutrients. There are three of them, namely protein, fat, and carbohydrates. Protein is required to build muscle while fat and carbs form the fuel for your body. Trying to work out and exercise without eating the right amount of carbs and fat is a bit like trying to drive a vehicle without any gas in it.

There is a lot of literature on proper nutrition partitioning and so on, but the best way to make sure you're eating the right amount of nutrients is to eat a balanced diet. This way, you're guaranteed to receive the right levels of nutrition.

Not Varying Your Workouts

I mentioned before that our bodies are incredibly adaptable and can adjust themselves to any workout or activity level over time. Once they adapt, they expend less energy in performing that activity. The result is that your rate of progress will slow down. The best way to avoid this is to switch your routines up and keep your body guessing.

There is the danger of going to the other extreme and varying your workouts too much. I'm not saying you should be doing something different every day, but an excellent way to determine when it's time to change is to monitor yourself for boredom. When you feel this coming on, change things, and charge your body again.

Lack of Tracking and Measurement

If you've worked out before, did you ever go to the gym with a notepad and a pen and keep track of how much and what you have lifted? Odds are you have never done this. This is pretty normal across all trainees. They assume that adopting a workout routine somehow guarantees they'll make progress and fail to realize that in order to progress, you need to measure and track performance. When you begin your workout session, you should know exactly what you're going to do as well as the duration and amount of time you'll be doing it for. Your training log contains all of this information, and you should be tracking everything you do. Think of it as being your progress log.

Poor Form

Many beginners rush into their workout routine full of energy and excitement and promptly injure themselves. This is because of them practicing improper form. Form here refers to the exercise technique. For example, if you're performing the pushup, you need to make sure your back remains straight and that it isn't bent. This is a straightforward instruction, but in a bid to squeeze that extra rep, some people are liable to bend their backs.

With bodyweight exercises, improper form will not result in massive injuries. However, this doesn't mean you should ignore form. Proper form ensures that you'll be building strength the right way and will be hitting the right muscles when you perform the exercise. Thus, in addition to preventing you from injuring yourself, form also guarantees a good level of strength and stamina.

Isolation too Soon

As I mentioned earlier, the huge guys at the gym tend to perform isolation exercises because it ties in with their goals (Why bodyweight training, 2019). Their goals happen to be very different from yours, and as such, it makes zero sense for you to follow their lead. Isolation exercises are best for those who are looking to give their muscles better shape.

They're not really geared towards building overall strength. For them to be effective, the trainee needs to possess a decent amount of muscle to begin with. At that stage, an isolation routine will help them develop both shape as well as help with their other lifts because it will ensure every muscle in the muscle chain is as strong as it can be.

Strength training is what gets your muscles talking to one another and working in tandem. It is pointless to strengthen one part of the chain when the chain itself barely exists. Hence, focus on the basics of strength first and worry about shape later. You'll look pretty good once you hit a decent level of strength, so don't worry about this.

What You Need to Succeed

Having covered the mistakes, a good question at this point is to ask what does one need in order to succeed? This is an extremely simple question to answer, thankfully. It comes down to two things:

- Patience and dedication
- Understanding the basics

Patience and Dedication

Rome wasn't built overnight, and neither will your strength and body be. On average, it takes around three months of consistent training for you to be able to see visible results in the mirror and for others to notice changes in you. If you feel three months are too far away, then understand that there is no magic pill or procedure you can undergo that will get you to where you want to go immediately. Life just doesn't work that way.

Besides, three months isn't really that long. Your first month will be spent getting used to your routine, and your second month is where you'll begin to start connecting things together. By the third month, exercise will become a habit for you, and you'll begin to feel the changes long before they appear in the mirror.

Things such as the difference in the way your clothes fit and your energy levels will make themselves known towards the end of the first month itself. The best way of looking at your routine is to break it down into a series of small tasks. By doing this, you'll prevent yourself from becoming overwhelmed and will be able to stay true to your course better.

Understanding the Basics

So how is strength built? How do your muscles grow? This process is a lot simpler than you can imagine. The amount of muscle mass in your body is referred to as your lean body mass. The higher your lean body mass is, the lower your body fat percentage. The greater your strength level is, the higher your lean body mass.

Thus, it's pretty simple: the more muscle you have, the less body fat you carry, and the stronger you are. When you exercise, your body is placed under stress. Now, you might think of stress as being a bad thing, but it's important to differentiate between good and bad versions of it.

Stress is terrible for us when it lasts for long periods of time. This is when your body starts producing hormones that disrupt your digestive system and place your brain on edge, ready to strike back against any perceived threats (Stoppler, 2018). When present for short durations, stress is good for us since it forces us to grow and learn new skills.

This is pretty much what exercise does. If you try to exercise for hours on end, you're going to be harming yourself. An ideal workout lasts for around an hour, followed by a nutritious meal within an hour of completing it. Post-workout nutrition is important because, during your exercise session, your body will be breaking down muscle fibers.

During your post-workout nutrition and resting period, you'll be providing your body with the fuel it needs to repair itself and grow stronger. Putting all of this together, the formula for muscle building is pretty straightforward: Focus on building strength, eat well, and rest well.

How This Book Will Work For You

Every exercise presented in this book is going to get you to build a basic level of strength before moving up a notch. One of the best ways to keep your body from adjusting to your current routine as well as to challenge itself continually is to keep adding new workouts that are aimed at increasing your strength level.

Thus, take the time to master a particular exercise prior to moving on to the next one. Do not be in a rush to try everything at once since this will result in you sabotaging yourself. Be patient and understand the basics. Review the common mistakes, and make sure you don't commit them.

It sounds simple, and in reality, it is. The key to success is often as simple as avoiding complicating things unnecessarily.

CHAPTER 2:

THE FOUNDATIONS OF
A HEALTHY LIFE

While exercise forms an integral part of a healthy lifestyle, it is just one part of it. If anything, exercise is only half the portion of it. This might sound surprising to you, but it is a fact (Carroll, 2015). There are three other things that are way more important for your health, and ensuring these are in order will go a long way towards good health.

In no particular order, these three things are:

1. Water
2. Sleep
3. Diet

This chapter is going to break down all of these three items, and by the end of it, you're going to know precisely what you need to do about all of them. Let's begin by looking at water first.

Water

The old adage that recommends drinking eight glasses of water per day is a useful metric to determine how much water you need to drink. However, keep in mind that this is a general piece of advice that is not meant to fit everybody's needs. As you've probably learned thus far, everyone's different.

Around 60% of the human body is made of water (Carroll, 2015). It is close to impossible to overstate how vital water is for healthy functioning. Water affects our body's processes right down to the cellular level, where it helps flush waste and re-energizes us. Water also plays a significant part in disposing of this waste via urine and sweat.

Speaking of sweat, water is what maintains your body's temperature at healthy levels. If you get too hot, sweat cools you down and ensures you don't melt from the inside (Carroll, 2015). In addition to this, water also plays a massive role in lubricating your joints and cushioning them. Layers of water around your sensitive organs protect them from harm as well.

These are just some of the ways in which water assists your overall health. One of the leading causes of poor health in the average American adult is dehydration. Dehydration occurs when you simply don't provide your body with enough water, and your body will immediately let you know when this occurs.

Some of the symptoms of dehydration are:

- Dizziness
- Headaches
- Lack of energy
- Inability to concentrate on tasks
- Tiredness or exhaustion

There are a few factors that go into determining how much water you need to drink every day. While the eight glass recommendation is a good place to begin with, depending on certain factors, you might discover that you need to drink a lot more.

Ideal Quantity

To figure out how much water you need to drink, we need to take a look at the factors that affect fluid levels in your body. The first and most obvious factor to look at is the climate you live in. Adult males living in temperate or pleasant climates require around 16 cups (four liters) of water, while adult females require 12 cups (three litres) per day.

The hotter the climate you're living in is, the more you're going to sweat, and you will need to replenish the fluid you lost. There's no way to calculate this accurately, but it's always better to increase the frequency at which you drink water the hotter it gets. The next factor that influences fluid intake is exercise.

The more you exercise, the more you sweat, and hence your need for water is higher. It is a good idea to drink a little water before your workout since this will energize you and ensure you don't dehydrate yourself in the middle of your workout. In between exercises, make it a habit to sip a little water. Once you're done, take a large swig of water as you rest and prepare to consume your post-workout meal.

I advise sticking to regular water instead of consuming fancy sports drinks. These drinks have their uses for people who work out for periods lasting longer than a couple of hours. When working out for this long, your body will lose electrolytes, and these drinks can help replenish them. However, for the purposes of the exercise program in this book, you don't need them.

Avoid consuming heavily caffeinated drinks before your workout since these dehydrate you to a greater extent than regular drinks. They will provide you with a nice kick of energy, but unless you're working out first thing in the morning, you don't need such stimulation.

Lastly, women who are pregnant or are breastfeeding should increase their fluid intake by at least two cups over the recommended intake amounts mentioned earlier (Gunnars, 2018). Monitor yourself for signs of dehydration and consult your doctor at all times.

How to Consume

You can consume water in multiple ways. First off, there is drinking, which is the most obvious way to do it. You can drink water or have any fluid, other than heavily caffeinated drinks. To make it clear, these drinks do contain water, but their calories come at a cost as you'll shortly learn. Don't consume them in excess.

Drinks such as milkshakes, smoothies, or juices contain ample amounts of water. If you're an avid juicer, you can consume juices of vegetables that contain high levels of water, such as leafy greens or cucumbers. Drinking juices of fruits, such as watermelon, is also an excellent way to get your daily dose of water.

Develop a routine around drinking water. Personally, I use a 40 oz flask to make sure I'm drinking the right amounts of water every day. I refill the flask at least three times, so I know that I'm drinking at least 120 oz per day (roughly just under a gallon of water). You can keep sipping from your flask throughout your day and monitor yourself for signs of inadequate fluid intake.

The signs to look out for are (Gunnars, 2018):

- Constantly feeling thirsty or hungry
- Urine is yellow in color or is not colorless

Thirst is sometimes confused as hunger, so always drink a little water when you feel hungry just to make sure you aren't getting your wires crossed. All in all, with a bit of discipline, you can ensure you'll never have to worry about your water intake throughout your day.

Too Much Water?

Is it possible to drink too much water? Technically yes. Excessive water consumption leads to a condition called hyponatremia (Gunnars, 2018). This occurs when your blood is heavily diluted to the extent where its sodium content is far too low. In such conditions, your kidneys cannot excrete the excess water.

Athletes who train for long periods of time are susceptible to this. Generally speaking, it is difficult for the average American adult to ever reach such levels of risk, so you probably don't need to worry about this.

Sleep

I've already mentioned in the previous chapter how vital the recovery period is for your progress. Indeed, your gains are made not during your workout but during your resting period. The most significant factor that affects the quality of your recovery is sleep. To be more precise, the quality of it.

Just like with water, the average adult requires at least eight hours of sleep every 24 hours (Roland, 2019). There are some exceptions of people who can get by with as little as six hours of sleep, but these people are truly rare. If you think you're one of them, odds are that you're underestimating your need for sleep.

The fact is that the average adult carries a significant sleep deficit. This is due to a variety of lifestyle factors. Furthermore, the type of lifestyle you lead also determines how much sleep you need. Some people actually require more than the customary eight hours. Let's take a look at what happens when we sleep before trying to figure out how much of it is needed.

Phases of Sleep

Sleep is often thought of as being a passive or inactive state. After all, all you need to do is lie there like a log and keep your eyes closed as your brain and body take care of everything else. While your body is at rest, the same is not true for your brain. If anything, it's just as active as it is when you're awake. The difference is the processes it carries out differ depending on the phase of sleep you're in.

There are two broad phases of sleep: Non REM and REM sleep. REM stands for Rapid Eye Movement. When you lie down to go to bed, you enter the non REM phase, which is subdivided into three stages. The first stage lasts for around 10 minutes and is characterized by light sleep, and you can be easily woken up at this time.

The second stage of non REM sleep lasts for close to 30 minutes and is when you slide deeper into slumber. You can be woken up at this stage, but it's a bit tougher to do so. The final stage is the longest lasting one and lasts for around 40 minutes or so. This is when your brain finally decides that the time is right to begin carrying out what it needs to do. Your blood pressure drops, as does your heart rate, and you begin to enter REM sleep.

REM, as the name suggests, is characterized by to and from eye movements underneath your eyelids. While in non REM mode, your brain is slowing things down, but here it picks the pace back up (Roland, 2019). Your heart rate and body temperature increase as your brain begins processing the things that happened during the day and begins embedding all the new skills you have learned.

In essence, this is the period when your brain is forming new neural pathways and is forging connections within itself. Research suggests that REM sleep is primarily concerned with restoring the brain and not so much the body (Roland, 2019).

When you sleep, you drift between periods of REM and non REM sleep. After the first period of REM sleep, you won't drift back into the first stage of non REM sleep but will hover around the second stage. This is why loud noises in the middle of the night can wake you up. Physical repair takes place during the non REM phase.

This is when human growth hormone or HGH is secreted, and this is used to repair your muscles and other soft tissue that has been placed under stress when exercising. HGH is what is responsible for muscle growth, and the only time it is present in the body in large quantities is during non REM sleep. Thus, skip on sleep, and you're not giving your body a chance to recover as it needs to.

Quality

It's tempting to think of sleep in terms of quantity and think that as long as you're logging in the hours, you're all right. This is a mistake. It's a bit like thinking that standing around in the gym doing nothing is going to cause muscle growth. There are a number of things that affect the quality of your sleep. The recommendation to sleep for eight hours assumes that those eight hours are high in quality.

If you exercise regularly or lead an active lifestyle, you need more than eight hours of sleep. The exact amount is not known, but an excellent way to get the ideal amount of sleep is to simply go to bed without setting your alarm. Wakeup whenever your body wants to the next day. If you have to wake up at a specific time, taking power naps throughout the day is a great way to boost productivity (Roland, 2019).

Ensuring total darkness in your bedroom and developing a sleep routine is essential to getting quality sleep. Limit the amount of time you stare into a bright screen such as your smartphone or a TV. Your brain will process the large quantity of light as being a cue to remain awake. Read a book as you lie down to start preparing your brain for sleep.

While white noise (regular and rhythmic noise at a low pitch) can help produce good quality sleep, you want to limit irregular noise since this has been proven to reduce sleep quality (Roland, 2019). You should ensure your bedding and pillows are of good quality as well.

Deficits

The reality of our busy schedules often makes it impossible to ensure high quality sleep at all times. This doesn't mean you should give up hope on ever sleeping well. One way to still receive your requisite hours is to take power naps during the day. These naps can be up to 30 minutes in length and will leave you feeling refreshed. It'll also help you avoid the mid-afternoon fog that affects people around 2:30-3 PM.

Another way is to go to bed on the weekends (or whenever you have a day off) without setting your alarm. Let your body and brain decide how much sleep you need. If you feel the need to sleep all day, so be it. It's not possible to completely overcome a large sleep deficit. What I mean is you can't stockpile a month's worth of lost sleep and then try to make up for it over the course of a week by not setting your alarm.

To overcome that deficit, you'll need to follow good sleep habits and make sure to develop a routine that will ensure as high a quality of sleep for you as possible. Lastly, develop some consistency around your sleep habits. In other words, go to bed and wake up at the same time every day. Your body will get used to this and will automatically begin shutting down during these times.

If you didn't sleep well during the night, get up at the same time in order to maintain consistency and try to make up for the lost sleep during the weekend. Prioritize sleep, and you'll find a lot of your problems related to fatigue and lethargy will disappear.

Diet

When it comes to fat loss and getting healthy, exercise is essential, but more than this, it is your diet that plays the most significant role. In fact, it is possible to lose fat without exercising, although I don't recommend this approach for the sake of your overall health.

If you think the fitness industry produces material that confuses people, this is nothing compared to what the diet industry does. There are all sorts of fancy diets out there that restrict one form of food and promote the other. These work to varying degrees. Truth be told, the majority of them are legitimate. This is mainly because eating healthy isn't rocket science.

Our bodies have an intuitive knowledge of what it needs to nourish ourselves. The problem is that we overcomplicate eating to the point where we end up confusing ourselves. The following tips will help you ensure you eat clean and maintain a healthy diet.

Choose Fresh

Always choose fresh and whole-food over refined and processed food. More than anything else, this will go a long way towards ensuring you eat healthily. Whole food refers to the stuff that exists in its natural form and is consumed with a little bit of cooking. Examples of whole food include grains, vegetables, meat, fruit, and so on. There is a school of thought that advocates eating food in a form that is closest to its natural state. This is generally good advice to follow, but there's no need to get fanatical about it.

Processed food can be a little confusing to get your head around at first. Technically speaking, anything that isn't present in nature is processed. For example, wine is processed, as is cheese. In moderate quantities, these aren't harmful. The types of processed foods you want to avoid at all costs are those that are chemically manipulated.

The food industry makes more money by producing stuff that lasts longer. To ensure this, they add chemicals and sugar that achieve this objective. The problem is that these chemicals wreak havoc on our internal organs and disrupt our digestive system. Anything that comes in a box, such as frozen pizza, fast food, TV dinners, and so on, should be avoided.

Meat and oil are two foods that suffer the most from processing. With meat, the processing usually occurs in the type of feed the animal is provided and the conditions it is housed in. Needless to say, most supermarket meat is sourced from farms that follow horrible practices (Myers, 2016). In some cases, livestock is fed plastic and other unnatural feed that results in all kinds of diseases being transferred to you when you consume them.

Oil is processed to ensure that it cooks better. A telltale sign of processed oil is its color. Natural, cold-pressed oil such as coconut or extra virgin olive oil is either not clear in color or tends to freeze quickly. In addition, they tend to be viscous. Processed oils have an almost watery texture and are clear in color.

Chemicals are added during the extraction process to squeeze the last bits of oil out of the husks of whatever the oil is being drawn from. For example, olive oil itself can be processed, which is why it is best to stick to extra virgin olive oil, as opposed to olive pomace oil, which is chemically processed.

Choose the Right Sugar

In addition to meat and oil, sugar comes in processed and unprocessed forms. Processed sugar is generally bad for you and is responsible for the majority of fat gains. Natural sugar, such as that found in fruits, honey and even in whole grains are naturally occurring carbohydrates and are important for your nutrition.

Choose natural sugar as much as possible. Having said that, remember that an excess of anything is bad. Just because natural sugar is good for you doesn't mean you can drink honey all day instead of water. Make sure your diet is balanced. Choosing whole grains and fresh fruits in your diet is the best way of making sure you receive the right quantities of this.

Eat Protein

Your muscles are literally made of protein, and the fact is that the average American diet is heavy in carbs and severely lacks protein. A good rule of thumb is to eat 0.7-1 grams of protein per pound of bodyweight. So if you weigh 200 pounds, you need to eat between 140 to 200 grams of protein as a part of your diet.

There are a number of healthy protein sources, both animal and plant-based. Animal sources tend to be denser and contain a higher concentration of protein within them. Plant-based sources usually contain a higher level of carbs along with protein. This isn't bad in any way. It's just that you might need to exercise at higher levels of intensity to burn the excess carbs.

Monitor Salt and Sugar

I've already mentioned sugar, but salt is something that most people ignore. They either consume too little or eat too much. The eating too much crowd usually ends up doing this by eating processed food, which happens to be high in sodium (i.e salt.) It's easy to eat too little by merely forgetting to add salt to the food you cook or not adding enough.

There's no need to overthink this. Add a few pinches of salt and monitor how much water your body is retaining. If you find that your stomach is full of water and you're constantly thirsty, you're probably overeating salt (as long as you aren't dehydrated.)

As for sugar, it is possible to eat too much of the right sort of sugar. Any excess carbs or sugar your body receives tends to get converted to fat, so you need to make sure you limit your consumption of it.

Break Your Meals Down

This is a contentious topic, but for beginners, it's best to eat multiple small meals throughout the day. This is because it keeps your blood sugar levels consistent, and you'll avoid experiencing the hunger spikes that occur when blood sugar levels drop. Be careful, though: it can be easy to overeat when doing this. Fix your meal portions ahead of time to minimize this risk.

Watch What You Drink

When planning your meals, it's easy to measure how much you eat, but most people forget to account for how much they drink. A cup of coffee here and a juice there adds up over the day, and you can easily consume more than 500 calories in this manner. It's best to stick to plain water if you want to drink something.

If drinking coffee, minimize the milk and sugar you add to it or even better, stick to herbal teas or green tea. Processed drinks such as Coca Cola and other assorted carbonated drinks only make things worse. Needless to say, alcohol of any kind guarantees you'll consume more calories than you need.

I'm not saying you should eliminate these things. Just minimize them while recognizing that elimination is the best option.

Exercise

All of us routinely eat more calories than we need. The best way to make sure we remain fit is to be physically active. Your bodyweight training routine will go a long way towards ensuring this but seek to be as active as possible. This means walking short distances instead of driving them. Take the stairs when you can instead of using the elevator.

Don't think of this as a routine. Simply make physical activity a part of your daily life, and you'll find yourself burning calories naturally. Furthermore, exercise makes you hungry, which is a sign that your body is burning what you give it efficiently.

Meal Prep

How would you like a method whereby you can guarantee that you'll always eat the right food in the right quantities? Meal prep is your answer! The way you choose to prep will be different from what someone else might decide to do. After all, your schedule determines how you'll go about doing this.

Many elements go into a good meal prep, so let's take a look at them one by one.

Storage

Figuring out food storage should be your first step. This is easy enough to do. You can buy plastic containers or glass bowls that you can use for this purpose. Storing food in plastic is not a great idea over the long term since the food will interact with it and produce harmful chemicals (Zandonella, 2010).

Storing your food in glassware is the best because of the lack of harmful byproducts and the fact that you can safely reheat your food in the bowl itself. In addition to this, you also want to refer to the United States Department of Agriculture guidelines about food storage safety. As a rule of thumb, don't aim to store food for more than three days in the fridge.

This means your cooking schedule is easy to figure out.

Cooking Schedule

If you're going to be storing food for three days at the most in your fridge, this means you'll be cooking twice a week. While the three-day rule applies to a lot of food, there are some items you can store for longer such as chopped vegetables, cooked beans, and so on.

A twice a week cooking schedule means you'll be cooking once over the weekend and once during the week. The weekday cooking session will need to be carried out efficiently if your schedule is packed. This is why it's a good idea to bake or slow cook your food. Take your time creating fancy dishes and recipes over the weekend.

I'm not saying your weekday cooked meals need to be lacking in flavor. It is entirely possible to cook food quickly and easily and still have it taste great. It's just a matter of learning how to cook.

Your Tools

If you're short on time to cook, one of the best things you can do is to focus on baking or slow cooking your dishes. This allows you to throw your food into the appliance and do something else while it cooks. The best part of this is that almost all types of food can be cooked in this manner. You can bake or slow cook meat, vegetables, grains etc.

Make sure you have the right tools to prep your food. This means having good quality knives, baking dishes and sheets, and a food processor. I recommend a food processor over a blender since this will enable you to do more than just a blender would.

Use Smart Recipes

Understand that the taste of your dish and the time it takes to create it have nothing to do with one another. A simple five-ingredient recipe that takes just 10 minutes to put together can be just as delicious as a recipe that has 20 ingredients and takes two hours to cook.

A great way to reduce your cooking time is to have smoothies or juices. This is especially true during breakfast time. A good lifehack is to add cocoa powder to any smoothie whose ingredients are less than appetizing to you. You can throw some protein such as eggs, milk, greens, avocado, peanut butter, or whatever strikes your fancy and have a readymade breakfast in no time.

If you feel hungry in between meals, consider carrying around trail mix or assorted nuts. These are packed with calories and will keep you full with a small helping. Focus on creating recipes that need simple cooking or baking and don't need multiple cooking methods in order to come together.

Salads are really easy to put together, generally speaking. You can prep the ingredients beforehand and store them in the fridge. If you're adding meat to it, you can choose to cook just this part of the recipe prior to consuming your meal.

Maintain Balance

The best way to create balanced meals is to ensure a variety of textures and colors on your plate. It seems absurd to suggest diversity in color, but this is one of the best ways to ensure you're eating a balanced meal. A simple formula of grain+protein+vegetables followed by a fruit-based snack or dessert almost always works.

Ensure you have a small helping of greens with your meals and you'll tick almost every box.

Meal prep doesn't need to be complicated. With a little planning and prioritization, you'll ensure that your meals will be tasty and delicious as well as healthy.

CHAPTER 3:

BODYWEIGHT TRAINING KNOWLEDGE: PROPER WARM-UP, STRETCHING, AND BREATHING

Now that we've covered some lifestyle basics, it's time to delve into the basics of bodyweight exercise. The good news is that you don't need any form of equipment other than a pullup bar. Even this is optional since what you basically need is a sturdy platform to hang from and pull yourself up. As you progress to more advanced calisthenics, you will need some equipment, but for now, a pullup bar is more than sufficient.

The rest of this chapter is going to give you everything you need to know about breathing, progression, frequency, and so on.

Workout Frequency and Other Concerns

When starting out, you should be working out three times a week with a day's gap in between workouts, as mentioned earlier. This is to give your body enough time to recover and also gives you the mental space to get adjusted to your workouts. Remember, the best kinds of trainings are ones that are as repeatable as possible.

If you were to rush headstrong into a new workout routine, your brain and body will rebel at the sudden change. Habit is a powerful thing, and if you're not accustomed to working out, your body isn't going to simply accept the new changes to its routine, no matter how excited or motivated you are.

Pretty soon, you'll find yourself becoming lazy or will develop mysterious 'injuries' that will cause you to miss workouts, and sure enough, you'll be back sitting on your couch in no time. Stick to the schedule mentioned above, and you'll be just fine. You might initially find this extremely easy and may not feel the 'burn' of a workout. This is intentional and allows your body to acclimate to the new routine slowly.

Where to Start

The chapters after this one will list the exercises you will need to perform. Each chapter will start by describing the easiest form of the exercise and will then proceed to more challenging forms. Every one arrives with differing strength levels, so it can be tough to figure out where you need to start exactly.

A good rule of thumb is to try all the versions of an exercise. When you find that you can do around four repetitions of an exercise variation, begin by performing the exercise that is one step lower. For example, the next chapter is all about pushups, and the progression is as follows:

- Incline Pushup
- Knee Pushup
- Pushups
- Diamond/Archer/Incline one arm Pushup
- One arm Pushup
- Weighted Pushup

Let's say you can perform four pushups. This means your starting level will be the knee pushup. You should do three sets of four reps of knee push-ups, to begin with. Performing four reps of the knee pushup counts as one set. You will perform one set, take a rest, and then perform another and so on until you complete three sets.

Rest Periods

How long should you rest between sets? Aim for an average rest period of one minute with a maximum of two minutes. Despite the word average, don't rest for 30 seconds after the first set and one minute thirty seconds after the second set. Keep your rest periods consistent, and you'll see progress. Do not rest for more than two minutes.

If you feel the need to do so, you're probably progressing too fast and need to take things down a notch.

Progression

When you begin, you'll be performing three sets of four reps per exercise variation. After the first day, you'll be resting for one day. The next session, aim to increase the first set by a single rep while keeping the remaining number of reps the same. For example, your pushup progression will look like the one below:

Workout day #1 - knee push ups (4,4,4)

Rest day

Workout day #2 - knee push ups(5,4,4)

Rest day

Workout day #3 - knee push ups (5,5,4)

Rest day

Workout day #4 - knee push ups (5,5,5)

Rest day

Workout day #5 - knee push ups (6,5,5)

And so on. You should aim to hit three sets of eight reps with each variation before moving onto the higher level. Sticking with our pushup example, once you can perform (8,8,8) of the knee pushup, your next workout will be to perform the pushup for (3,3,3). Aim to increase your reps in the same manner.

Don't try to shortcut this process by adding more than one rep for the reasons mentioned earlier with regard to how your body adjusts to your new routine. Take it slow, and you'll find yourself making greater progress in the long run.

Shortcuts

I'll keep this one simple: There are none. You need to perform every rep in the full range of motion without trying to shortcut progress. Any rep that you cannot perform with the full range of motion doesn't count as a valid rep. Don't take a breather of 10 seconds in between a set to get the last rep out. Keep your cadence as consistent as possible.

Cadence

Speaking of cadence, you should spend two seconds in the concentric phase and three seconds on the eccentric phase. Concentric phases are the ones where you're tensing your muscles, and eccentric is when you're releasing the pressure. In a pushup, the concentric phase is when you go down towards the floor, and the eccentric phase is when you push off the floor (Cross, 2018).

You should pause for about a second in between phases.

Stalling

With this program, stalling should not be a major concern. If you follow the progression as outlined, you'll find that moving from (8,8,8) to (4,4,4) of the higher level should come easily. Sometimes, it is possible that the next level is too tough, and you cannot complete (4,4,4). In such instances, increase the number of reps at the lower progression to 12 and try again.

In other words, if you find yourself unable to complete (4,4,4), go down one level and aim to increase your reps to (12,12,12) from (8,8,8.) This will generally fix all problems. If you're still unable to complete (4,4,4) of the higher progression, aim for (3,3,3) and start from there.

Another form of stalling that occurs is within the current level itself. For example, you might find yourself unable to progress beyond (7,7,7) for whatever reason. A single session's worth of a lack of progress doesn't count as a stall. If you find yourself unable to progress beyond three sessions, deload the number of reps you're performing.

This means you'll perform (6,6,6) during the next session and then work your way back up to (7,7,7). This applies to all rep combinations. For example, if you were stuck at (7,7,6), you'll still deload to (6,6,6) and work your way back up. Another good idea is to monitor your rest and recovery periods. You want to feel fresh and ready to go prior to your workout. If you're exhausted just thinking about it, take an additional rest day and come back refreshed.

Imbalances

You'll eventually progress to one arm exercise variations, and these will present a challenge. Almost everyone has some form of strength imbalance, and you'll find that you'll be able to perform more reps on one side than the other. To eliminate this, begin with your weak side first and perform the same number of reps on your stronger side, even if you can do more.

Warm-Ups

A great workout routine starts with a great warm-up. As I mentioned previously, warm-ups are something we innately understand and yet fail to implement when it comes to exercising. I'm not sure what the reasons for this are, and it's unimportant to get into all of it. Suffice to say that you should be warming up no matter what.

An excellent warm-up reduces your risk of injury by heating your body's temperature to a certain point (Cross, 2018). Warm muscles are more pliable and are more responsive to stimulation. In practical terms, this means you're going to perform better, and you'll have reduced soreness post-workout.

Soreness is something you'll have to deal with in the beginning since your body isn't used to the activity you're subjecting it to. This makes it even more critical for you to prepare your body before a workout. A good warmup ensures that your body is prepared for the more strenuous movement that is to follow, and it also gets you mentally prepared for your workout.

So with this being said, let's look at the best warmup routine you should implement prior to your workouts.

Step #1 - Jump or Skip Rope

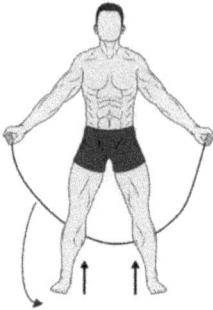

Skipping a rope has long been used as an effective warmup by not just bodybuilders but also by athletes and boxers. It gets the blood flowing and also helps with your coordination. If you cannot skip a rope to save your life, you can jump in the same spot, run in the same place or do jumping jacks.

Run on the spot or skip rope for 5 minutes.

Step #2 - Shoulder Rotations

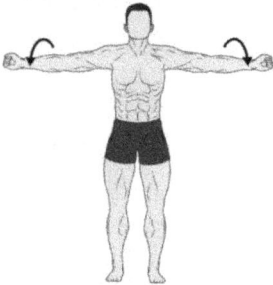

Opening up your joints is extremely important, and shoulder rotations do the job admirably. The exercise is pretty simple. Simply rotate both of your arms backwards in a controlled manner. You can move them forward as well if that's more comfortable for you. Alternatively, you can do one arm at a time.

Perform 5 shoulder rotations per arm.

Step #3 - Arm Raises

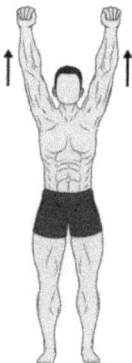

This exercise also focuses on loosening your shoulder joints. Simply raise your arms above your head and swing them up and down in a controlled manner. You don't want to exercise your power here while swinging. Just focus on how your shoulder moves and focus on the increased sense of warmth as blood flows through it.

Perform 5 arm raises for both arms.

Step #4 - Torso Twists

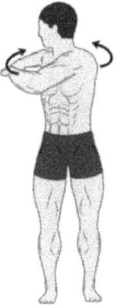

From the shoulders, we now move to the hips. Twist your core to the left and right in a controlled manner. As you twist, notice how your lower back feels. You can try to tighten your core as you reach the extremity of your twist.

Perform 5 torso twists. Remember that one twist to the left and right counts as a single twist.

Step #5 - Chest Expansion

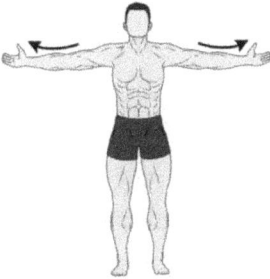

Your chest is one of the biggest muscles in your body and is more of a muscle chain than a single muscle. It comprises pretty much all of your upper body, so loosening this up is essential if you want to perform well in your workout. Place your arms by your side; bring them up and out as you expand your chest.

Perform 5 chest expansions with palms facing upwards.

Step #6 - Neck Rotations

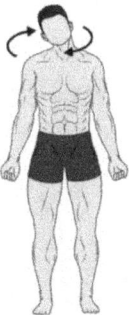

Your neck contains important muscles that stabilize your head. When exercising, these muscles receive an automatic workout, and if they're not warmed up properly, it can lead to sprains and other unwanted things. Simply rotate your head in a clockwise or counterclockwise direction.

Perform 5 to the left and 5 to the right.

Step #7 - Hip Rotation

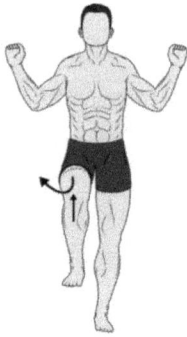

Thanks to sitting down all day, your hips are probably locked shut. The hip joint is one of the most flexible in the body and has a wide range of motion. This exercise unlocks it. Adopt a staggered stance, much like a boxer would. Lift your back leg off the ground and rotate your hip in order to bring it forward. This is a single rotation.

Perform 5 hip rotations on each leg.

Step #8 - Reverse Hip Rotation

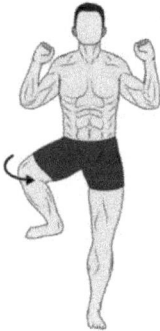

Once the previous exercise is done, rotate your hips in the opposite direction from the same stance. In the previous exercise, you brought your leg forward. Now rotate your hip backwards to loosen them up even more.

Perform 5 reverse hip rotations on each leg.

Step #9 - Leg Swing

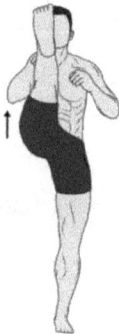

From a standing position, place your right arm out in front of you. Now, raise your right leg out front until it reaches the level of your extended arm. Bring your leg up in a controlled manner. This is a raise and not a kick. Having said that, you don't need to bring it up too slowly. Experiment with what speed works best for you and focus on loosening your hips and your hamstrings.

Perform 5 leg swings per leg.

Loosening your hips is extremely important, and if you feel that they're still not warmed up properly, you can perform a couple of variations of the leg swing. Hold onto a vertical frame of some kind at arm's length and stand next to it. Your arm will thus be extended out to your side. Swing the leg that is farthest away from the frame back and forth. Repeat this with the other leg.

Now face the frame and place both hands on it, with your torso bent at a roughly 60 degree angle. Swing your left leg from side to side while keeping your torso as straight as possible. Repeat with the right leg.

Post Workout Routine

Don't be alarmed by reading the name of this section. There are no additional exercises for you to perform once you're done. Instead, you'll need to begin stretching after your workout in order to start your recovery process. A lot of people ignore this portion of their workout, including experienced trainees.

The fact is that post-workout stretches play an essential role in recovery. You'll be less sore the following days and will feel more relaxed once done. Let's look at some of the benefits of an excellent post-workout stretching routine.

Flexibility

Strength is not measured just by the amount of muscle you have but also by how flexible that muscle is. While mass generates power, flexibility is what ensures that the muscle is pliable and won't give in when stressed in uncommon ways. During your workout, your muscles are going to be packed together in order to generate power.

Loosening them up improves flexibility and also improves your performance for your next workout by enhancing the recovery process.

Blood Circulation

Once a muscle tenses up, blood flow into it is constricted. In addition to this, your heart will pump at a higher rate, and your body overall is under quite a lot of stress. Stretching while cooling down improves blood circulation. Recovery begins when oxygen-rich blood begins to flow through your muscles. This enables the cells in your muscle tissues to repair themselves and become stronger.

Lactic Acid

As your muscles are stressed, the oxygen within them depletes since your body is going to be using all the oxygen it can get its hands on. This leads to the formation of lactic acid, which gradually increases as you workout. One of the things that increases the rate at which lactic acid is dissipated is increased blood flow.

Stretching achieves this goal by enhancing blood flow through your muscles, and thus, the damage caused by lactic acid production is reduced significantly.

Energy Boost

As your body cools down, your brain releases endorphins. These chemicals are commonly known as 'feel good' chemicals and are what energize you after a workout. Stretching speeds up the recovery process, and thus endorphin production occurs at a faster rate. As a result, you feel energized and ready to go sooner.

Pain Minimization

Sore and tight muscles often lead to injury. Stretching after a workout reduces the risk of this by loosening them up and minimizing any pain you might feel.

Better Coordination

Stretching your muscles after a workout has been shown to increase their functional mobility (Cross, 2018). One of the reasons this occurs is because your muscles are forced to relax together as you stretch and, thus, learn to work in tandem better. The result is that they synchronize better, and your effective strength increases.

Mind-Body Connection

Stretching helps slow the body down gradually instead of abruptly stopping it after a workout. Stretching involves a lot of slow breathing and observation of your muscles. This increases the connection your mind has with your body, and you'll become more aware of what's going on within you.

The result is an increased sense of peace and awareness and a better mood overall. Now that you understand the benefits of stretching post workout, let's look at the routine itself.

Your Post Workout Routine

Follow this step by step post-workout stretch routine to maximize your recovery. Hold these poses for 12 seconds in order to return the muscles to their original length. You can hold the poses for up to 20 seconds in order to increase flexibility.

Step #1 Pectorals Stretch

Stand a few feet ahead of a pole or any vertical frame you can hold. Stretch one hand back with your palm facing up and push your hand against the frame in order to stretch your upper chest. Repeat the motion with the other arm.

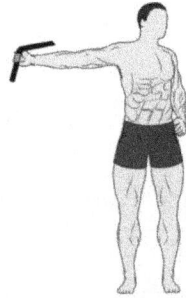

Step #2 Lats Stretch

Stand in front of a wall a few feet away, and raise one hand up, palm fully open. Place it on the wall and press yourself towards the wall gently. Repeat with the other arm.

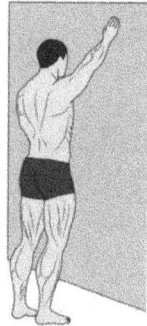

Step #3 Triceps and Lats Stretch

Raise your arms up and bend them at the elbow behind your head. Using the fingers of one hand, gently pull the elbow of the other arm inwards until you feel a stretch in the tricep muscle. Repeat with the other arm.

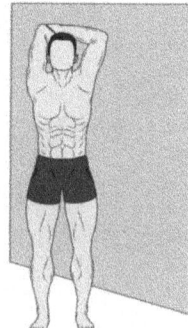

Step #4 Pecs and Rotator Cuff Stretch

Place your forearms flat on either side of a doorway and lean forward gently.

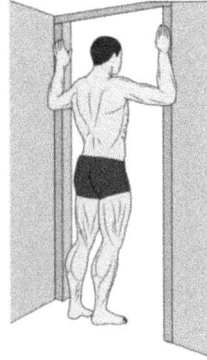

Step #5 Calf Stretch

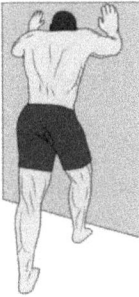

Stand a few feet away from a wall facing it and lean forward to place your palms on the wall with one leg ahead of the other. Repeat with the other leg.

Step #6 Calf Stretch #2

From the same position as the previous exercise, place your back leg on its toe and gently bend your front knee towards the wall. Repeat with the other leg.

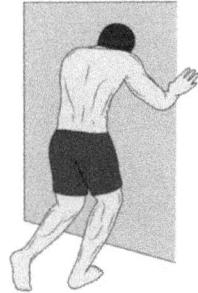

Step #7 Quad Stretch

Stand on one leg and bend the other leg backwards at the knee until you can grip your toes. Pull the toes to increase the stretch. Repeat with the other leg.

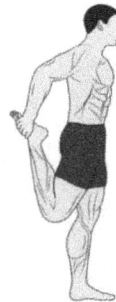

Step #8 Hamstring Stretch

Place one leg on a bench with your leg straight. Without bending your knee, lean forward as much as you can. Repeat with the other leg.

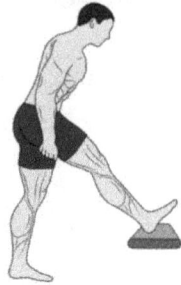

Step #9 Hamstrings and Adductor Stretch

Rotate 90 degrees to the outside from the previous position and bed sideways towards the bench. Repeat with the other leg.

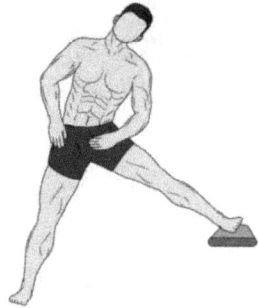

Step #10 Adductor Stretch

Stand with your legs wide apart and bend forward as low as you can.

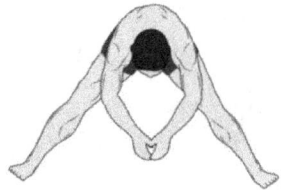

Step #11 Adductors and Calf Stretch

Sit on your heels and squat as low as you can. Place your elbows on the inside of your knees and push your knees outwards.

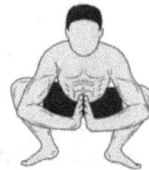

Step #12 Glute Stretch

Sit on the floor and bend one leg 90 degrees at the knee. Simultaneously lift the other leg and place it on the outside of the knee of the bent leg. Repeat with the other leg.

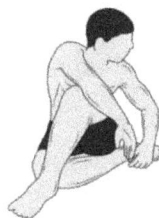

Step #13 Cobra Stretch

Lay down on the floor on your belly and raise your chest off the floor with your palms planted firmly on the floor.

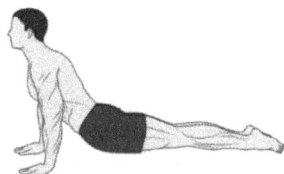

Step #14 Cat Stretch

Place yourself on all fours on your knees and palms. Make sure your head is in line between your palms. Now, bend your neck forward while rounding your upper back.

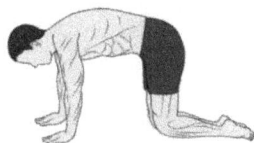

Breathing

One of the most basic things you can do to guarantee better performance and to ensure you don't suffer from injuries is to breathe properly. Breathing is something many beginners don't pay attention to and understandably so. They focus on proper form and the weight they need to lift and forget that breathing well is a part of the equation.

Breathing not only oxygenates your blood, but it also helps firm your body up against stress. If your body isn't firm during the right time when exercising, you're liable to injure yourself. Figuring out when to breathe isn't all that complicated. Always remember to breathe out during the exertion phase of an exercise.

For example, on the pushup, the exertion phase is when you push yourself off the ground. This means you breathe in on the way down and exhale as you push up. In a pull-up, the exertion phase is when you're pulling yourself up and breathing in is when you lower yourself down. So you inhale on the way down and exhale on the way up.

One of the other advantages of breathing correctly is that as your blood becomes more oxygenated, it burns fat and carbs more efficiently. In other words, not only does your body fuel itself better, but it also burns fat faster. Additional weight loss is also realized thanks to the body being able to excrete excess water and toxins better under such conditions.

So always remember to breathe correctly. Perform your exercises slowly at first to get used to the breathing rhythm, and as time goes by, you'll adjust to it.

PART 2

FUNDAMENTAL
EXERCISES

CHAPTER 4:
MASTERING THE PUSH - PROGRESSIONS FOR THE PUSHUP

The first exercise you're going to learn is the pushup. This is a versatile exercise and has long been considered a barometer for upper body strength. The pushup engages not just your upper body but your core and lower body as well. Your arms, chest, and shoulders work to stabilize and push you off the ground. Your core ensures you don't twist and bend your back while your lower body works to make sure you remain stable.

The best part about the pushup is that you can modify it easily to suit your strength level quickly and easily. There is no end to the number of variations of a pushup since you can modify both the speed as well as the form of your pushup. Let's begin by looking at the classic pushup and the form you must hold to perform it well.

Pushup Form

For a simple exercise, it's startling to see how many people get this basic movement all wrong. Aside from the reasons mentioned earlier about how form plays a vital role in determining progress, proper pushup form allows you to evaluate your strength from session to session accurately. If you were to perform one session with perfect form and the other with poor form, there's no way of knowing your true strength level.

Let's break down the various elements of pushup form one by one.

Hand Position

Your hands should be placed slightly wider than shoulder-width apart. This is a step that a lot of people get wrong, and they tend to place their arms too wide. This results in flared elbows when they go down and push themselves back up. Think of it this way: when looking at your body from above, you should look like an arrow, not like a T with your arms out to the side.

Wrists

Your wrists need to be flexible to do a proper pushup. This isn't the case for a lot of people. If this applies to you or if your wrists hurt when performing the exercise, you can use bars to grasp. These will reduce the pressure on your wrists. Alternatively, you can perform them on softer ground such as grass or dirt.

Another modification you can make here is to clench your palms into fists and place these on the ground. These clenched fist pushups will hurt at first so you can build up to them by performing them on soft surfaces first and gradually increase the degree of difficulty. Although I recommend you starting with open hands with palms touching the floor, perform easier variations, and slowly your wrists will become stronger and stronger.

Feet

Your feet should be out behind you in a position that is most comfortable for you. You can place them wide or close together, the choice is entirely yours, and there's no single right way to do this. Generally speaking, the wider your feet are, the more stable your base will be, but to gain the most benefits, always have your feet together and knees straight so your body looks like a pencil.

Core

An essential part of pushup form is to make sure your backside isn't sticking up in the air. This happens when your lower back hinges at the hips. A good way to ensure this never happens is to tighten your glutes (backside) and abs and think of your entire body from toe to head as being one single unit. A tip is to tighten every muscle in your core and legs straight. As you lower and raise your body, be aware of your back's position at all times.

Some people tend to bend their upper back as well by rounding it. Again, contracting your abs makes sure this will never happen.

Head

As you push up and down, your head should be looking slightly down and not straight ahead. Looking ahead will place your head out of alignment with the rest of your torso, and this will likely strain your neck muscles. Simply look slightly down and not straight ahead.

Elbows

At the top of your pushup, you want your arms to be straight, but you should not lock your elbows. Locking your elbows will just leave you in an awkward position, so don't do this.

All of these points might seem like there's a lot to remember. The best way to practice this is to place yourself into the pushup position and then gently lower and raise yourself as you practice all of these points. One of the things that makes push-ups so easy to get wrong is that they're challenging to practice consciously. What I mean is that it's pretty tricky to hold your position at the top and then lower yourself slowly as you think about your form as well.

The best way to monitor this is to film yourself as you perform a pushup. Setup a camera off to the side or have a friend film you. Don't forget to film yourself from above as well since you want to make sure your elbows are not flaring out. When performing the regular pushup, you don't want your elbows to flare. This is not the case with some of the more advanced variations, such as the one-armed pushup, as you'll see later in this chapter.

Performing the push up from this position is pretty straightforward. With your glutes and abs tight, lower yourself gently. Don't do this slowly at first since you'll exhaust yourself. You can take around two seconds to lower yourself. The lowest point is different for everyone. A good rule of thumb is to have your elbows bent at 90 degrees or as close to it as possible.

At this point, either your nose or your chest will be touching the ground. Make sure you repeat the movement as consistently as you can so that you're measuring the same move repeatedly. Don't measure one rep as your nose touching the ground and the next with your chest and so on. Consistency is key here.

Take special care to keep your elbows tucked. Don't tuck them in deliberately, but just make sure they don't flare out. This usually happens when you begin to get tired and can't raise yourself anymore. Flaring elbows will cause injuries to your shoulders and wrists, so avoid this when performing the standard pushup.

The push up might be a standard exercise, but this doesn't mean everyone can perform it by default. A lot of people struggle with it, and if you find that you can't perform a single rep, then you need to start at lower levels and work your way up as detailed previously. The way to do this is to practice incline pushups and then knee push-ups. Let's take a look at them one by one.

Easier Variations

These two variations of the pushup will enable you to strengthen your upper body muscles in preparation for a regular pushup. Remember that the objective here is to strengthen your upper body with a view to performing the pushup down the road. So don't get too comfortable with these exercises since they aren't the ultimate objective.

The first variation we'll look at is the knee pushup.

Pushup Progression

As mentioned earlier, all exercises in this book range from the level of a novice to an expert. I've already described how to find your ideal starting point and work forward from there. If you happen to start from the knee pushup level, you'll progress from there to the incline pushup. From there, you'll progress to the regular pushup. Once you can perform (8,8,8) on the regular pushup, you will need to take things up a notch.

Knee Pushups

To begin the knee pushup, kneel down and roll your body forward until you're supporting yourself on all fours. You might want to roll your torso forward a little to reduce the load on your kneecaps. If they hurt, you can place a cushion under them or perform the push up on a soft ground.

Gently lower yourself by bending your elbows. Go as low as you can go and then push up through the palms of your hands. Throughout this movement, make sure you observe proper form as outlined previously.

While clenching your glutes is less important here since you're kneeling, you should make sure your back remains straight. Do not arch or round your back since this takes the load off your shoulders and also forces your body into an unnatural position. Begin by performing three sets of four reps (4,4,4) as previously outlined and follow the progression.

You can place your palms slightly wider than shoulder-width when performing this pushup. As with every other pushup variation, you can change the difficulty level and the muscles hit by modifying the placement of your palms. Place them close together, and you'll place greater strain on your biceps and triceps.

Place them far apart, and you'll engage your upper back and chest more. The shoulder-width stance is a good in-between place to engage both sets of muscles optimally.

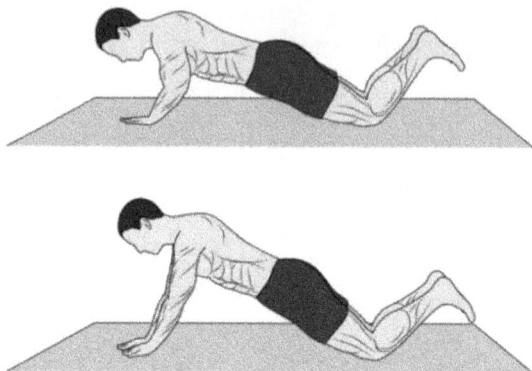

Begin by doing 3 sets of 4 reps (4,4,4). Work your way up to 3 sets of 8 reps to move on to the next progression (8,8,8).

Incline Pushups

Incline pushups are one level up from knee push ups. In other words, once you're able to complete (8,8,8) of knee push ups, you should progress to inclines. You can think of incline pushups as having the same technique as regular pushups but performed with your hands on an elevated platform instead of on the floor.

To begin, kneel down and extend your arms forward until they're on a bench or some elevated platform. You can place your hands on your bed as well. With your arms fully extended, lift your knees off the ground and clench your glutes and abs. Your body should be a straight line from your heel to the crown of your head.

Gently lower yourself onto the bench (or whatever platform you're using) and push yourself up until your arms are straight. Perform the rep progressions as indicated previously. You will need to pay more attention to your form here than with knee push ups.

The first thing to look for is the placement of your elbows. Don't allow them to flare outwards and do not lock them at the top of your motion. Do not round your back and don't stare down. In other words, you need to follow the same form tips as with a regular pushup.

An additional concern here is the platform you're using. Make sure it's stable and that it won't slide out in front of you. This will result in you falling flat on your face and you might sustain an injury. As with the knee pushup, you can adjust the placement of your elbows to place stress on different parts of your upper body. As recommended earlier, keep it simple and place your palms at a little more than shoulder width apart.

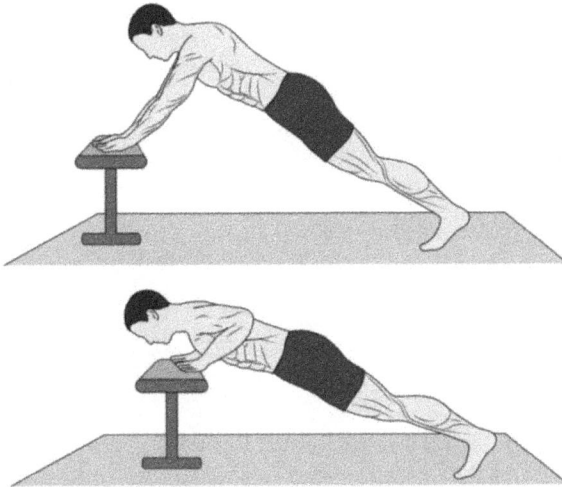

Begin by doing 3 sets of 4 reps (4,4,4). Work your way up to 3 sets of 8 reps to move on to the next progression (8,8,8).

Basic Pushup

The form for this has been explained already. Place your arms slightly outside your shoulder and lower yourself. Now exhale as you push yourself off the ground. Make sure your elbows are tucked in and your core remains tight.

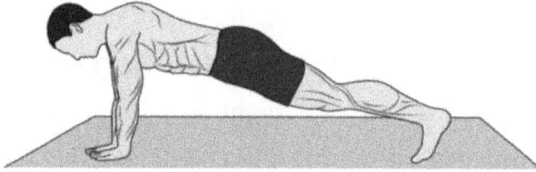

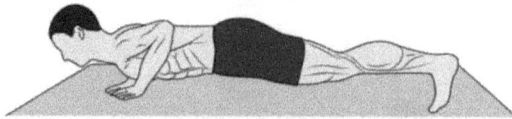

Begin by doing 3 sets of 4 reps (4,4,4). Work your way up to 3 sets of 8 reps to move on to the next progression (8,8,8).

Diamond Pushup

The form for the diamond pushup is exactly the same as a regular pushup except for the placement of your palms. In this variation, you'll place your palms close together, right underneath your chin, and form a diamond-shaped pattern with your hands. The index fingers from both hands will touch one another as will your two thumbs. This results in a diamond shape, which gives the variation its name.

To perform the push-up, lower and raise yourself as you would with a regular pushup. Diamond pushups are a lot harder on the biceps and triceps and don't engage the chest as much as the regular variation does. As such, these are pretty difficult to perform so don't be afraid to take your time with them.

A variation you can introduce here if you find the step from a regular pushup to a diamond too steep is to do the knee pushup with a diamond grip to help you out on those final few reps. These don't officially count towards your progress, but it can help you achieve some mental satisfaction and reduce your fatigue in the moment.

Either way, follow the same progression and training pattern when performing this and be careful of flaring your elbows out wide.

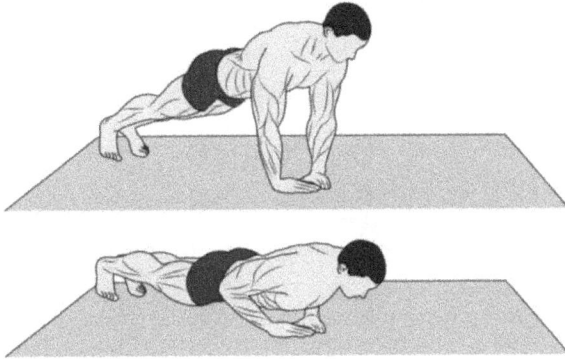

Begin by doing 3 sets of 4 reps (4,4,4). Work your way up to 3 sets of 8 reps to move on to the next progression (8,8,8).

Archer Pushup

The Archer is a step above the diamond pushup. This variation prepares you for the next level, the one armed pushup, which is extremely tough to perform. Finding your ideal starting point with the Archer pushup takes some time, so be patient with it. The form is exactly the same as with a regular pushup except for your hand placement.

In the Archer, you'll be placing one arm out straight in a position where it doesn't help with your pushup. How far you choose to place it depends on your comfort level. The further out your hand is, the tougher the exercise will be. You need to find a balance between your comfort level and toughness. In other words, you want to be comfortable enough to perform a few reps of the exercise, but don't make it so easy that it doesn't vary from a regular pushup all that much.

Lower yourself on one arm and push back up while making sure your torso is straight and that your elbows aren't flaring out to the side. Look forward and not directly underneath you in order to maintain a straight line from your ankles to your head. The Archer is a tough variation to perform, so here are a few things you can do to enhance your performance.

Tighten everything. From your toes to your glutes to your abs, your chest, your back, whatever else you can think of, tighten it. Tightening everything ensures you won't suffer from an injury and also ensures that you won't have to waste energy trying to make up for something else that's sagging behind you, such as your hips or belly. This way, your energy can be concentrated in your upper body where it's needed the most.

Remember to breathe properly at all times. As you do this, you might find your breath steps out of sync with your push up. In such cases, simply abandon the set and try again.

As you push up, push through your armpit and not your shoulder. This will help you engage your lats better and will add additional force to your movement. A variation of the Archer you can try is to place your other hand out to the side on a dumbbell or a slightly raised surface. This makes the exercise a lot harder and will build your strength.

Once you've done all of this, repeat it on the other arm!

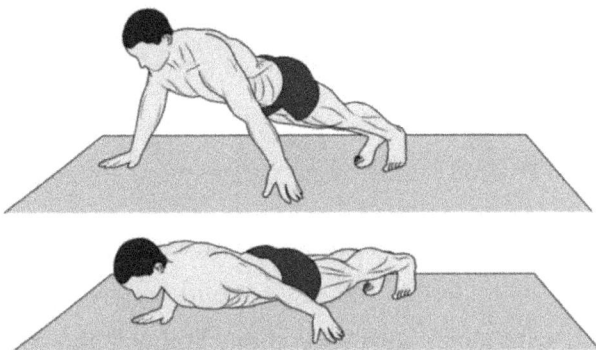

Begin by doing 3 sets of 4 reps (4,4,4). Work your way up to 3 sets of 8 reps to move on to the next progression (8,8,8).

Incline One Arm Pushup

These are exactly the same as incline pushups, but you'll be doing them with one arm instead of two. Place your arm slightly outside your shoulder and lower yourself. Now push up off the bench to complete the movement. Make sure your elbow doesn't flare out too much to the side and you keep your hips in line with your spine. Repeat with the other arm.

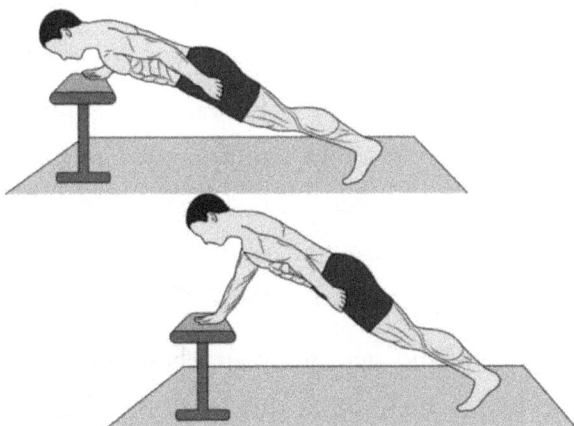

Begin by doing 3 sets of 4 reps (4,4,4). Work your way up to 3 sets of 8 reps to move on to the next progression (8,8,8).

One Arm Pushups (OAPs)

The one-arm pushup is the ultimate form when it comes to pushup progression. It will build serious strength in your upper back, shoulders, and arms along with your chest. You will also develop a solid core since you will need to stabilize yourself. As with everything else, it is best to follow a progression on OAPs as well.

The first level is the incline OAP. Tuck one arm behind your back and press downwards into the bench or platform. You can go as low as you feel comfortable going. Generally, this level is when your elbow is bent at a 90-degree angle. Take care to maintain a steady torso angle and don't slip sideways by opening your chest too much.

The next level is the negative OAP, where you focus only on the decline portion of the exercise on the floor. In other words, you lower yourself down, and that's it. Don't try to push yourself back up. Doing this increases your awareness about your core and lets you know the optimal level for your lowest position on the pushup. You can push yourself up with both arms once you've gone down.

The third level is the wide arm OAP, also called the Rocky variation after the movie of the same name. This variation requires you to flare your working elbow out wide. In addition to this, your opposite leg will also be placed wide in order to provide greater stability. Keep your biceps parallel to the floor and your elbow at a 90-degree angle as you flat it out wide at the top of your position.

Lower yourself down and activate your chest muscles as you push yourself up. I'd like to mention at this point that flaring your elbows out wide in this position is not harmful for you. The issue arises when you place your hands close to your torso and flare your elbows. This results in a rotation of the shoulders that is unhealthy.

In the Rocky pushup, you're placing your arm out wide, and as such, there is no danger of injury. The next level of progression is the decline OAP where you place your feet on an elevated surface and lower yourself. Given that your feet are at an incline, this makes pushing up incredibly difficult. The rewards are worth it though.

The final and highest level of progression is the single-leg OAP. In this, you lift the leg on the working side up. Thus, your support will be along a diagonal line between your working arm and the leg on your nonworking side. You can place your arm out wide or close to you as you desire. By the time you reach this level, you'll probably know yourself enough to understand what works best for you.

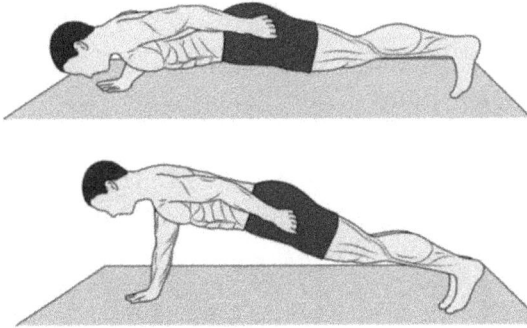

Begin by doing 3 sets of 4 reps (4,4,4). Work your way up to 3 sets of 8 reps to move on to the next progression (8,8,8).

General Progression Option

You're free to follow the progression as indicated, or you can alternatively choose to weigh your pushups. The best way to do this is to wear a weighted vest and increase the weight gradually. This allows for a longer progression cycle since you can keep increasing the weight infinitely.

Ideally, you can explore weighted pushups once you can perform some form of a one-handed pushup. The decline and one-legged OAP are both pretty tough, and the weighted pushup is a good option at this point. If you don't have access to a weighted vest, you can place some form of weight on your upper back. The problem with this approach is that the weight is likely to slide off you, and unless you have access to barbell plates, you cannot measure the weight accurately.

However, if you wish to take this option, it is a great one to increase your strength.

CHAPTER 5:

THE PERFECT PISTOLS: ACHIEVING PERFECT FORM FOR SUPERIOR LEGS

Leg day is synonymous with torture in the regular gym-going circles. Odes have been written to this mythical day when the average gym-goer prepares to go through hell. I might be exaggerating a little bit, but there's no doubt that training your legs is not an easy task. There are a few reasons for this. The first is that our leg muscles comprise a significant amount of our overall muscle mass.

Training such a large group of muscles requires a lot of effort and time. This brings me to the second point as to why training your legs is hard. We use them to support ourselves throughout the day and after our workout. If you've just trained your legs, it isn't uncommon to feel as if you can't support your weight anymore.

This is quite normal and is just a feeling. In other words, your legs are more than capable of holding you up no matter how much you train them in this program. So don't worry about collapsing. While you won't be able to run up a flight of stairs, walking about will be perfectly possible.

When it comes to bodyweight training for your legs, there's just one exercise you need to master: The squat.

Squats

Squats are the king of all exercises. Everyone from Olympic athletes to bodybuilders to regular gym trainees accept this as a fact. There's a very good reason for this. Squats are often thought of as being a leg movement but are, in fact, a total body movement. There isn't any other exercise that will work out every single muscle in your body like the squat can.

Your legs bear the primary load that you will carry during squats. The rest of your body assists in lifting the load and stabilizes it, but it is your legs that will drive the weight up and down. In our case, the weight is simply your body weight. Bodyweight squats are a basic form of exercise, and you should seek to master them before even thinking about adding additional weight.

The reason is that the squat is an extremely technical exercise and is practically worthless if not performed with proper form. Even worse, squatting with heavyweight and improper form leads to pretty bad injuries. This is not a concern for you; however, you shouldn't assume this to be a free pass to squat incorrectly.

A lot of people can squat but few squat well. There are a lot of myths surrounding the squat, so let's take some time to clear these up as well as look at the benefits of a good squat.

Natural Motion

In the Western world, we aren't accustomed to squatting and tend to think of the movement as being bad for our knees. However, travel to the less developed parts of the world, and you'll find loads of people squatting all the way down, with their knees fully bent and their backsides near their ankles.

The fact is that the human body is designed to squat, and the movement signifies a certain level of fitness. This is because, in order to squat all the way down (bodybuilders refer to this as ATG- Ass to Grass), you need to be flexible. Your hips need to be unlocked fully, your knees need to be loose enough to bend fully, your core needs to be strong enough to balance you, your lower back needs to be stable enough to support your core, and your ankles need to be flexible enough to bend.

Squats are also a traditional resting position and relax your body a lot more than sitting down does. This is because a full squat (with your hands around your knees) allows you to hold yourself and exhale and inhale better. Thus, you'll find that your lungs fill with air more efficiently, and you won't be out of breath for so long.

Not to mention the fact that if there are no chairs around, you can still sit and relax.

Versatility

I've already mentioned how the squat trains every part of your body. It demands both strength and flexibility. It develops core strength and makes your lower back stronger. The lower back is an area that is often left untouched or is trained incorrectly by most people. When trying to train the lower back, most people perform stretches and bend over. This does train the lower back to a certain extent, but its true purpose isn't to stretch (Hadim, 2012).

Instead, the lower back is needed to stabilize you along with your core. Thus, the best way to train it is to place it under heavy loads, and to have it remain stable. Squats, when performed with weights or with bodyweight, does this job perfectly. As you squat down, your lower back needs to remain stable while supporting your upper body.

Simultaneously, your core is pushing in from the front and assisting your lower back. This develops the muscle communication process within your core and builds the mind and body connection.

Joint Training

While your muscles contribute quite a lot to your overall flexibility, your joints are the ones that do the heavy lifting. When you perform a bodyweight squat, your hips, knees, and ankles are tested and strengthened. There is a lot of misinformation with regard to squats and knee health.

You will often hear a lot of people recommend against performing the squat thanks to the possibility of knee injuries. This is a bit like saying you should never drive since you could end up in a fatal accident. It doesn't depend on the nature of driving as much as in the way you drive. With squats, your form is everything.

Contrary to the myth, squats actually strengthen your knees and hips (Hadim, 2012). When performed correctly, your knees are forced to remain stable, and the muscles around it are strengthened. Your hips are forced into their full range of motion, and as a result, you'll find that once you are squatting well, you'll feel looser in that part of your body.

Your ankles are also strengthened thanks to the load they need to bear and remain stable. The only joint missing from all of this is your shoulder. However, when you perform squats with a bar, your wrists and shoulders are also tested. Don't worry about this for now since we're solely focused on bodyweight squats.

Squat Form

So now that we've looked at the benefits, it's time to look at what makes a great squat. Being a full-body exercise, it will take some time for you to fully come to grips with all the things you need to do. As you read these points, take the time to practice your form. You won't get it right the first time.

It's best to video yourself and take pictures of your form to get feedback on how you're doing.

1. Stand up with your feet around shoulder-width apart. To improve your balance, keep your feet pointed slightly towards the outside.

2. Keep your neck in a neutral position, and don't lock it. Your gaze should be fixed ahead of you and will move in a straight line up and down as you lower and raise yourself. Pick a spot that's at eye level or slightly below it.

3. Extend your hands out in front of you or touch your shoulders with the opposite arm, so you can touch your right shoulder with your left arm and left shoulder with your right. As your arms bend, they will create a platform. Take a deep breath and inhale air into your diaphragm (not your belly). Contract your abdomen in and tighten your abs.

4. Now comes the tough bit. The key to squatting is to bend through your hips, not your knees. The way to do this is to sit back.

5. Extend your hips backward and gently lower yourself. If you don't know what a hip extension feels like, think of it as lowering yourself onto a chair. Except, keep your arms and chest up.

6. Your knees should remain in the same position, and it will be fine if it moves forward a bit. They will bend, of course, but

during the descent should they come ahead of your toes slightly.

7. Your weight when you descend should be on your heels. You might feel as if you're about to fall backward, but don't worry. This will not happen unless you deliberately try to do so.

8. Remember to keep your chest big and arms up at all times!

9. As you descend, aim to break parallel. This means your hips should be lower than your knees and your thighs will be at a slight angle to the ground. Don't aim to go all the way down at first. Simply break parallel.

10. A squat isn't a squat unless you break parallel!

11. Hold your position at the bottom for a beat. Now, it's time to rise back up.

12. With your belly still pushed in and chest up, tighten your glutes. Your glutes are extremely powerful muscles, and once fully activated, you'll find that they can literally throw you out of the bottom position.

13. Keep your chest up and abs contracted to stabilize your core. If your chest isn't up, you'll find that your knees will roll forward.

14. Raise your hips and chest together. What you will experience at first is that your glutes will push your hips up, but your chest will lag. With some practice and video feedback, this will correct itself. Think of your torso as being one block. Raise it upwards at the same time.

15. Raise yourself up to a standing position.

16. Repeat!

That's a lot of steps you need to follow, but don't worry about not being able to master them. With repeated practice, it'll become second nature to you.

Achieving Flexibility

To perform deep squats, you need to be flexible. Some people just aren't as flexible as others are, and with this in mind, the following warm-up routine will get you primed to squat as deeply as possible. Perform this routine regularly, and you'll find yourself becoming more flexible as time goes by.

1. Loosen your hips by performing the exercises listed in the warm-up routine two chapters ago. The leg swings help with this the most.

2. Squatting, by itself, is a great way to loosen your muscles. Simply squat as low as you can. You'll feel your hamstrings stretch when you do this. Don't look to raise yourself out of this position. You might even find that your back rounds. This is fine as long as you're not placing any major load on it.

3. From this deep position, bring your right knee to your left toes and your left knee to your right toes.

4. Next, stretch your right leg out to the side and maintain your balance on your left foot as best as you can. This stretches your right leg out nicely.

5. Repeat the motion with your other leg.

6. Stand up and place your legs wide apart from one another. Maintaining this position, reach as far forward as you can while keeping your knees straight.

7. Stand up and rotate your ankles to loosen them up.

8. Perform a few more leg swings if you still feel tightness in your hips.

Squat Progression

Find your ideal starting point, as mentioned in the earlier chapter. Work your way through the progression in the same way as you would through the pushups. Begin by completing (4,4,4) of these and then progress to the next level once you complete (8,8,8.)

Assisted Squats

You can use a chair for an assisted squat. To begin, place a chair in front of you with its back towards you.

Place your hands on the top of the chair and squat down with proper form. Remember to keep your chest up, and as you ascend, make sure you squeeze your glutes. Follow the same form as detailed with regard to the squat previously. Keep your chest up at all times and squeeze your abs in as you ascend.

Avoid using the chair to propel yourself upwards too much. In other words, don't use your arms to push yourself up or to stabilize you too much as you descend or ascend. Think of it as providing support instead of it being a prop to push yourself up or lower yourself.

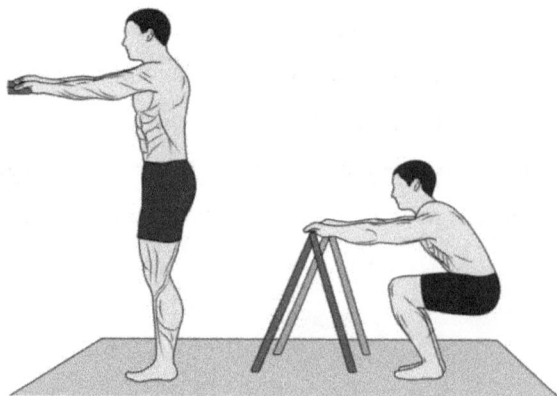

Begin by doing 3 sets of 4 reps (4,4,4). Work your way up to 3 sets of 8 reps to move on to the next progression (8,8,8).

Deep Assisted Squats

These are the same as the previous exercise except for the depth at which you'll be squatting. In the previous exercise, you'll be breaking parallel, but here you'll be squatting all the way down with your knees fully bent.

In other words, assume the same form as in the previous progression but squat all the way down until your bottom is almost touching the floor and your knees are fully bent.

When coming back up, make sure you don't use the assistance off the chair too much to pull yourself up. Keep your abs tight and chest up and look straight ahead (as opposed to upwards.)

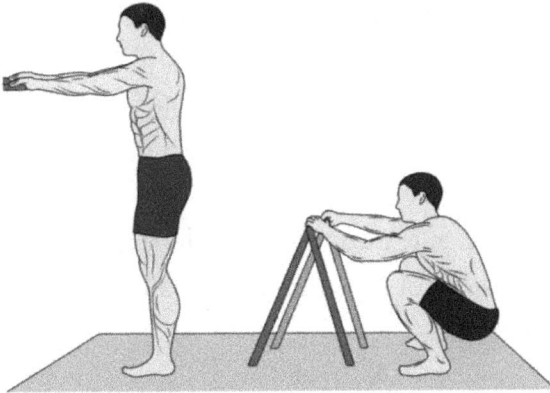

Begin by doing 3 sets of 4 reps (4,4,4). Work your way up to 3 sets of 8 reps to move on to the next progression (8,8,8).

Squats

This is the proper squat. Descend until your thighs are parallel with the floor. When lowering yourself, monitor your back to make sure it doesn't round. A symptom of your back rounding is when your lower back sinks inwards towards your knees. Follow the form discussed earlier in this chapter.

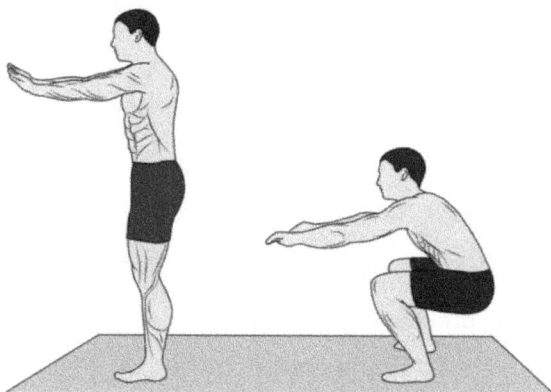

Begin by doing 3 sets of 4 reps (4,4,4). Work your way up to 3 sets of 8 reps to move on to the next progression (8,8,8).

Deep Squats

Same as the previous one, except here you'll be going all the way down. In other words, instead of squatting past parallel, you'll be going all the way down to the ground.

A particular problem most beginners have here is with regard to their back rounding when they move below parallel. Keep your chest up and abs tight and descend past parallel as slowly as you can. A sign of back rounding is when your lower back dips inwards towards your knees at the bottom.

You can film yourself to make sure your form is correct and ensure you aren't rounding. As always, remember to look straight ahead and not up.

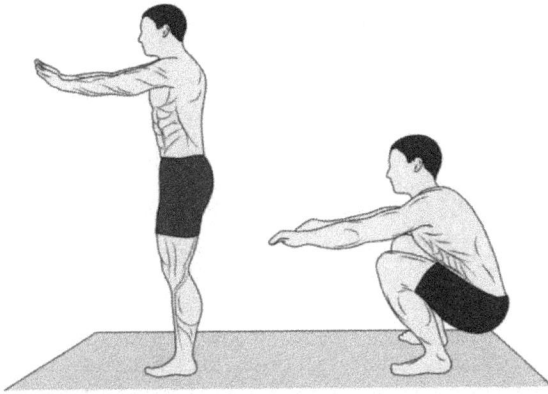

Begin by doing 3 sets of 4 reps (4,4,4). Work your way up to 3 sets of 8 reps to move on to the next progression (8,8,8).

Closed Squats

Place your feet close together until they're touching one another. Now squat as you normally would by extending your hips backwards. In this variation, you'll find that your upper back will round a bit. This is fine. Take care to not round it too much though, since this is harmful in the long run.

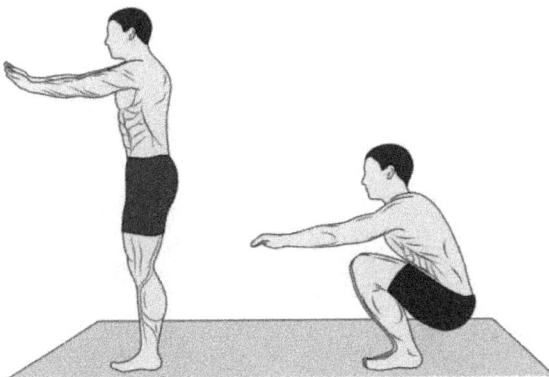

Begin by doing 3 sets of 4 reps (4,4,4). Work your way up to 3 sets of 8 reps to move on to the next progression (8,8,8).

Bulgarian Split Squats

Place a platform or bench behind you. Now, extend one foot back and place your foot on the platform with the sole of your foot pointing upwards. Extend your back foot as much as possible by moving forward. Make sure your front thigh is perpendicular to the floor. This is the starting position.

Gently lower yourself and try to get your back knee to touch the floor or get as close to it as possible. Make sure your back foot is still in contact with the bench behind you. It will take some time to find the ideal spacing for this, so take your time with it and don't rush the process.

When lifting yourself back up, remember to squeeze your front glutes to propel yourself upwards. Keep your abs tight throughout the routine.

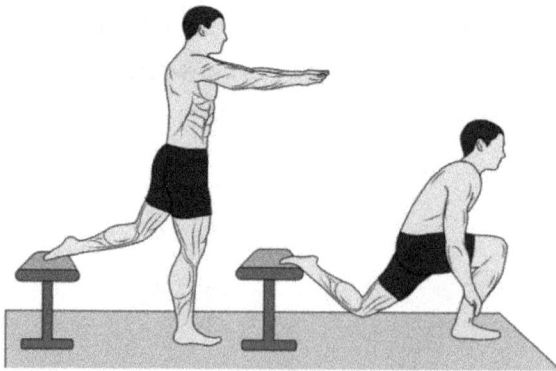

Begin by doing 3 sets of 4 reps (4,4,4). Work your way up to 3 sets of 8 reps to move on to the next progression (8,8,8).

Shrimp Squats

Remove the bench from the previous exercise and squat with your back leg in the air. Lower yourself to the floor until your back knee and toes touch the floor at the same time. In other words, the lower part of your extended back leg should be straight.

Make sure you descend in a straight line and don't overbalance out to the sides too much. Keep your abs tight and look straight ahead as you ascend and descend.

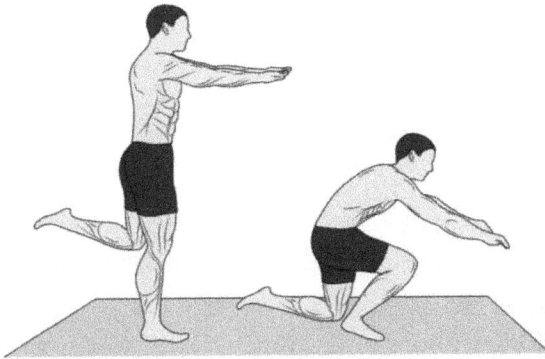

Begin by doing 3 sets of 4 reps (4,4,4). Work your way up to 3 sets of 8 reps to move on to the next progression (8,8,8).

Assisted One-Legged Squats

Place a bench or a chair next to you. Now, stretch one leg out in front of you and one arm out in front to stabilize yourself.

Lower yourself until your backside touches the back of the heel of the foot that is not extended. You can use the bench to push yourself back up by applying pressure on it with your hand. Make sure your back heel remains flat on the floor, and your front leg remains elevated.

Repeat the routine on the other leg as well.

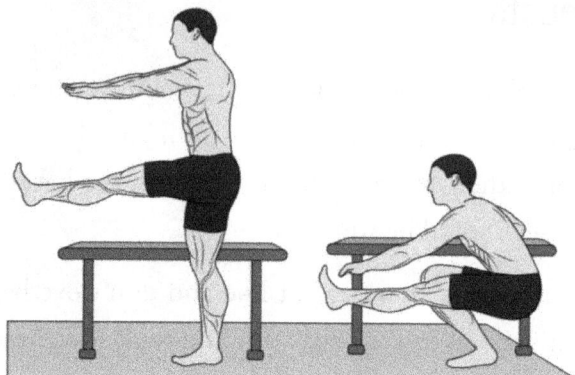

Begin by doing 3 sets of 4 reps (4,4,4). Work your way up to 3 sets of 8 reps to move on to the next progression (8,8,8).

Pistol Squats

These are unassisted one-legged squats. Make sure your arms are extended out in front of you. Descend on one leg with the other extended out in front of you. Follow the same tips here as in the previous step. Your shoulders should be in a neutral position, and you should not roll them forward as you ascend.

If you do this, your back rounds, and this is something you want to avoid with squats. Also, make sure you don't move your torso ahead of your knees when descending since this is improper form.

Descend and ascend in a controlled manner and tighten your core at all times to maintain stability.

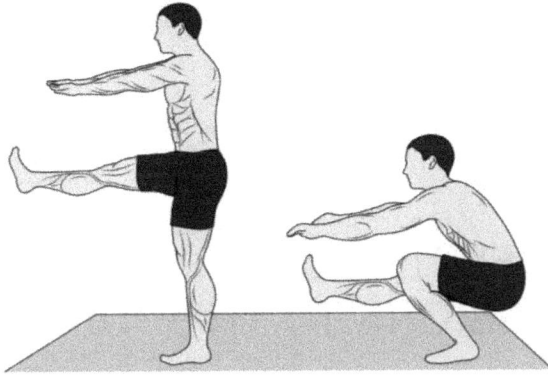

Begin by doing 3 sets of 4 reps (4,4,4). Work your way up to 3 sets of 8 reps to move on to the next progression (8,8,8).

CHAPTER 6:

THE PERFECT PULLUP: PROGRESSIONS TO THE PULLUP

The pullup is perhaps the second most popular bodyweight exercise along with the pushup. Just as with the pushup, the pullup is an essential component of your workout regime, and the better you get at this, the better your overall performance will be. The primary muscles targeted in the pullup are your back and shoulders, along with your core receiving some secondary benefits.

As with the pushup, there are many variations you can implement with the pullup to make it even more potent. You can add a variation that targets your back a lot more and another that works your arms out.

Pullups

Beginners to strength training often fail to grasp how in-tune your entire body is and how a balance exists within it. For example, your core has two sides to it: Your front core, which is comprised of your abs, and your rear core, which is your lower back. Similarly, your upper body has two large chains of muscles that work to support it at all times.

The chain of chest and arm muscles stabilize the front while the back muscles work the rear. Generally speaking, every training program has to have a balance in terms of training the front and back. Without this, imbalances develop. For example, if you have an imbalance where your chest is a lot stronger than your back, you'll find that your shoulders will roll forward since the back isn't strong enough to pull them back into position.

Thus, as tempting as it might seem to choose to perform just the pullup or just the pushup, you need to focus equally on both for optimum performance. Finding a balance between exercises can be as simple as looking at the motion that is being carried out in them. The push up requires you to push while the pull up requires you to pull. It really is that simple. Having a good balance between your exercise motions will ensure you'll grow strong evenly.

Benefits

The chain of muscles in your back is even more intricate than the chest muscles in the front. The back muscle chain comprises of your lats, scapular retractors, and the upper back muscles. All of these work together to help you move and lift weight, and it can be tough to train all of them at once.

The pullup is one of the few exercises that trains all of them together. The only other exercise that is comparable to this is the deadlift, and that requires you to lift a weight off the floor and is not a bodyweight exercise.

The back muscles aren't just all about strength. They also play a significant role in your posture. Given that they exist on the other side of the shoulder joint, your back muscles work to stabilize your body up top. Poor posture often leads to injuries that are brought about by muscle imbalances. Furthermore, strength in the body that is in balance will lead to healthier shoulder blades and a healthier body.

Speaking of the shoulder, the pull up trains your shoulder heads as well. You can perform a variation of the exercise to target the trapezius muscles that exist just below the back of your neck. Performing the pullup well also results in your performance on your other lifts, increasing it proportionally. This is because a lot of the muscles used in those exercises are used in the pullup.

Lastly, the pullup is often used as a standard gauge of strength by armed forces all around the world. It's pretty easy to see where you rank by comparing your performance to the standards demanded by them.

How to do Them

Like the pushup, the pull up looks simple to perform, but people still manage to practice it with improper form and don't do themselves any favors. The first thing to do is to get yourself either a pullup bar or find something you can grab onto to pull yourself. This can be a metal rod or a wooden beam of some sort. Although the shower curtain rod does not count!

If there's nothing at home, you can check out a playground or a park that has an outdoor gym. Famous beaches often have pull up bars that you can use. Grab the bar overhead and hang from it. Pull yourself up until your chin passes the bar and lower yourself. That's pretty much all there is to it. Make sure you follow the points below with regards to your form.

1. Begin by paying attention to your grip - Your palms should face away from you and should be shoulder-width apart. You can modify your grip to change the muscles targeted. Holding your hands close together and having your palms face, one another will target your arms. A wide grip will target your lats and back a lot more. For now, keep them shoulder-width apart.

2. You will be hanging, to begin with - You can bend your knees or let them hang if you have space below. Take care not to bend your knees and then use them to give yourself a jerk upwards. You should keep your legs as still as possible. Take care to start the hang by making your body a dead weight.

3. Now deeply inhale and pull yourself upwards!- Like with the pushup, make sure your elbows are tucked in and don't flare outwards. Doing this shortens the distance you need to travel and will also result in an injury. So, avoid doing this.

4. As you pull yourself up, make your chest big and as you raise yourself, try to touch the bar with it.

5. Remember to breathe and exhale during the ascent! This might become difficult as you progress. In such cases, breathe in on the way down and exhale on the way up.

6. When pulling, think of the motion as being one where you're pulling your elbows down and bringing your shoulder blades together, as opposed to one where you're pulling yourself up by the shoulders. Lead with your chest on the way up.

7. At the top - Make sure your chin goes above the bar or else it doesn't count. When lowering yourself, make sure you extend your arms fully. Don't lock your elbows at the bottom.

Here are some other things to keep in mind:

1. Head - Keep a neutral position and don't try to reach forward. Don't end up headbutting the bar in your enthusiasm to get up there. Look ahead, and don't tilt your head at any angle.

2. Lower back - Arching your back will give you a bit of a boost, but don't do this. Over time, you'll weaken your back and will sustain an injury.

3. Shoulders - It might seem tempting to do this at the top, but don't squeeze your shoulder blades together too much.

4. Thumbs - Curl your thumbs around the bar and grip it as hard as you can. This will activate your muscles more. The bar should rest at the point where your fingers meet your palm.
5. Palms - One variation of the pullup is referred to as a chin up. The only difference between the two is the grip. In a chin up, you'll hold the bar with your palms facing you.

Pullup Progressions

If you cannot do a single pullup or think that you're far too heavy to be able to do pull ups successfully, think again. These progressions will help you build your strength up to a point where you can perform pull ups efficiently. As for being too heavy, the issue isn't your weight as much as it is to do with your lack of strength. Keep working out, and you'll have no problems with pullups. But also, keep in mind the less fat you have, the easier this exercise will be.

Leg Assisted Pullups

If you've ever been to a gym, you've probably seen the assisted pullup machine. This machine has a platform that you can stand on, and this pushes you up and down as you pull on the overhead bar. This exercise is a home version of it. Stand on a chair and grab onto the overhead bar.

As you pull, lift one leg off the chair and curl it like you would on a standard pullup. Use the other leg to push yourself and assist with the process. The great thing about this variation is that you can choose your exact level of assistance as well as modify it over time. Needless to say, you want to keep reducing the level of assistance you receive and begin using your upper body to pull yourself up.

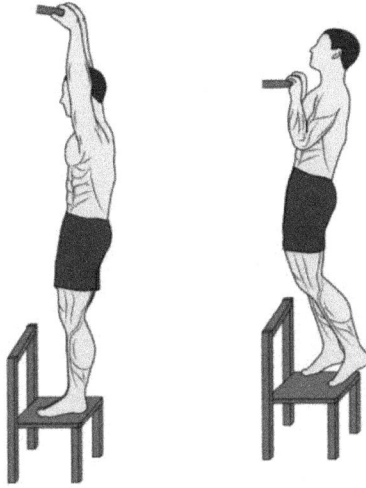

Begin by doing 3 sets of 4 reps (4,4,4). Work your way up to 3 sets of 8 reps to move on to the next progression (8,8,8).

Jackknife Pullups

Jackknifes are a bit tricky to get right. The way they work is like this: place a chair or a platform far enough away from you so that you can rest your heels on top of it. Grip the overhead bar and rest your feet on the platform in front of you. Perform a pullup as you usually would. This is a tough progression, and you might find that you'll need to begin with (3,3,3) instead of (4,4,4.)

Don't lose hope or get discouraged. Pullups are harder to progress through than pushups, and for this reason, you need to be patient.

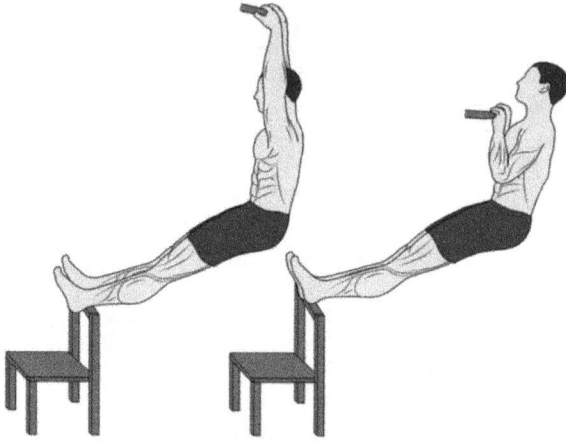

Begin by doing 3 sets of 4 reps (4,4,4). Work your way up to 3 sets of 8 reps to move on to the next progression (8,8,8).

Half Pullups

As the name suggests, this is a half pullup. Raise yourself to a level equal to the midpoint of a full pullup. Your arms should be bent around 90 degrees at this point. From this point, raise yourself upwards until your chin is above the bar. Do not use any assistance to do this.

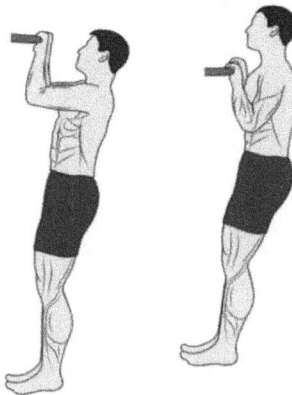

Begin by doing 3 sets of 4 reps (4,4,4). Work your way up to 3 sets of 8 reps to move on to the next progression (8,8,8).

Pullups

The full exercise, as described at the beginning of this chapter.

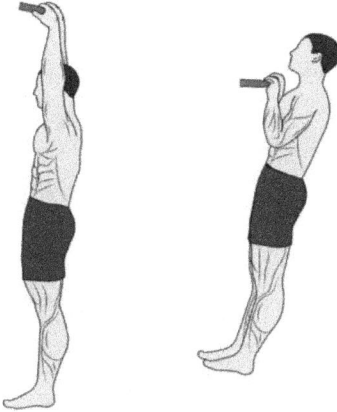

Begin by doing 3 sets of 4 reps (4,4,4). Work your way up to 3 sets of 8 reps to move on to the next progression (8,8,8).

Close Grip Pullups

As mentioned earlier, this variation places a lot more emphasis on your arms. Bring your hands closer together on the bar. You can place them as close as you'd like. Ideally, the thumbs of both hands should be touching one another.

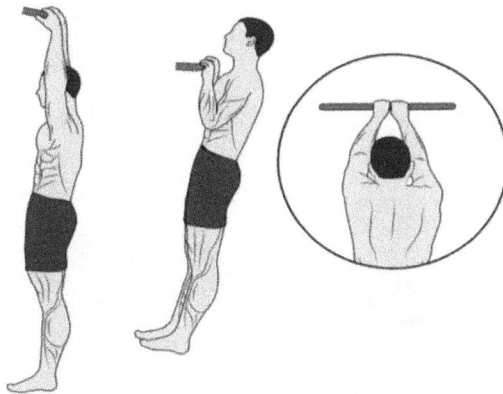

Begin by doing 3 sets of 4 reps (4,4,4). Work your way up to 3 sets of 8 reps to move on to the next progression (8,8,8).

Wide Grip Pullups

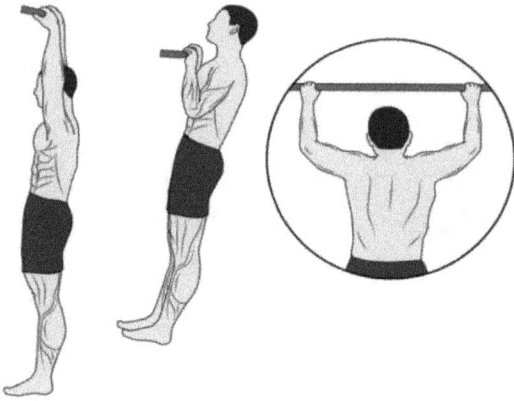

Place your hands out wide and lift yourself up. The range of motion on the variation is shorter. You'll find that your back will be worked a lot more.

Begin by doing 3 sets of 4 reps (4,4,4). Work your way up to 3 sets of 8 reps to move on to the next progression (8,8,8).

Archer Pullups

Yup, Archer exists with pullups as well. To do these, begin by using one arm to a greater degree to pull yourself up. Over time, keep moving the other arm out wider until it is fully extended. The aim is to be able to pull yourself up with one arm, with a bit of assistance from the other. With the Archer, it's important to alternate pull between both arms.

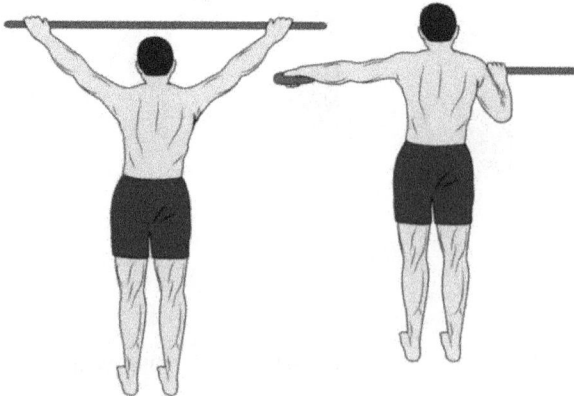

Also, the maximum number of reps you should aim for here is six. So aim for (6,6,6) before progressing.

CHAPTER 7:
A SIX PACK OF STEEL: LEG RAISES

Let's face it. One of the reasons you want to get fit is to be able to rock a six pack. Well, the best way to gain a six pack is by performing a leg raise. Aside from cosmetic purposes, there are many reasons you want to have a strong core. In this chapter, you're going to learn how your core muscles work to keep you stable and fit and why you should care about them beyond purely visual purposes.

The Core

To understand why leg raises are so efficient at building a great core, we need to take a step back and examine how any muscle is developed. As I mentioned earlier in the section on exercise basics, there are two types of training you can engage in. The first is to perform a compound movement that recruits a large number of muscles, and exercises in this category closely resemble tasks you'll carry out in real life.

For example, the squat is a compound movement that tests and trains a large number of muscles throughout your body. It helps you perform movements in real life as well as develops your overall flexibility. This is perhaps the biggest positives of compound movements. Not only do they help you build muscle, but they also make those muscles flexible since the entire muscle chain is developed.

The second type of training is referred to as isolation training. As the name suggests, this involves training a muscle in isolation and concentrating all your effort into moving just that muscle. For example, curling your arms with a weight at the end of each is an isolation exercise aimed at increasing the size of your biceps.

Isolation exercises don't develop the muscle chain, and with this, any strength gains that they bring make the muscle a little less flexible. This is why beginners don't benefit from isolation training. If the muscle chain is not well developed in the trainee, the isolated muscle has no way of expressing its strength. It simply doesn't know how to talk to the muscles surrounding it, and this results in dangerous strength imbalances.

Isolation exercises do have their place, but it isn't in a beginner's workout routine. As I mentioned earlier, the perfect time to begin implementing isolation routines is when you've already developed a base level of strength. The best way to increase your strength is to perform compound movements that recruit as many muscles as possible.

So what is the best compound movement to train your abdominals?

Ab Training

Your core muscles, which include your abdominals, are tasked with a number of functions. First, they need to maintain your posture and keep you from simply falling over. Your front abdominals and lower back work hard to prevent this from happening. Next, below your abs is another layer of muscle that is far more important. This muscle acts like a band around your body and keeps your internal organs in place.

It also plays a vital role in breathing and helps you exhale forcefully should the need ever arise. Thus, without the abdominals doing their thing, you're likely to run into several issues. This is why fitness is a lot more than just having six pack abs. A six pack isn't much of an indicator of fitness at all. It merely means that the person with it understands the importance of low body fat in conjunction with abs.

All compound movements train your abs to a certain degree. The squat, pushup, and pullup need you to maintain a stable torso, and thus your abs will be trained on a secondary basis. Whether you can see your abs or not is a function of how much fat you're carrying around your midsection. This area of our bodies is where most of us carry the majority of our fat.

In men, it most certainly is where the most substantial amount of fat collects while in women, the midsection and butt are where fat resides. Understand that there is no way to laser target fat via exercise. Losing fat is a function of eating healthy, in the right amounts, and building muscle. Do these three, and fat loss will take care of itself. Performing a million crunches is not going to help you develop your abs or get them to show themselves any more than walking will.

Crunches are an example of an isolation exercise that doesn't do much for beginners. You can crunch away all you want, but if your entire abdominal chain isn't developed, there's not much the exercise is going to do. The best way to train your abs is to perform exercises that target the spinal column and place stress on it.

Training in general, and all exercises in this book, do this automatically. However, leg raises focus on maintaining spinal stability under stress and therefore are just the ticket when you're looking to train your core. By performing them well, you'll develop a strong core, and a six pack will become inevitable. Once you've developed initial strength in your core, feel free to do as many crunches as you want. Understand that isolation exercises on your core will only give them better definition. You're not going to grow new abs all of a sudden by doing them.

The leg raise is a fundamental movement that can be done pretty much anywhere. You need a bar to hang from, which can be your pullup bar or some beam you use to pull yourself up. One of the great things about leg raises is that they work the obliques as well, which are the core muscles on the side of your abs. Since your spine stretches during the movement, you'll be training the muscles that are responsible for spinal stability as well.

Throughout the movement, your lower back needs to be stable, and this further strengthens it. The flip side of all this is that leg raises are not an easy exercise to execute. Almost everyone, even experienced trainees, will begin near the bottom half of the progression simply because most people don't train their abs using compound movements.

Form

The leg raise, or hanging leg raise as it's more commonly called, has many variants. The purest form requires you to hang from a pullup bar and lift your legs straight up and curl your pelvis up until your toes touch your fingers. The key to working your core with every version of the leg raise is to tilt your pelvis upwards. Your pelvis is the bone that accompanies your hip joint.

An easy method of making sure you're doing this is to place a mirror in front of you. When you perform a raise of any kind, make sure you can see your backside come upwards as you lift your legs. If you cannot see your backside, you're not fully engaging your core.

One of the variations that a lot of experienced trainees use is to bend their knees and lift them up to their shoulders. This is a step below the straight-legged hanging leg raise and also works your core out strenuously. Whatever the variation, remember to keep your chest balanced and don't try to exaggerate its position.

Another thing to keep in mind when hanging is that you will need to engage your shoulders a little as you raise your legs upwards. Some variations include suspending straps and delegating the hanging bit to these. This reduces the degree to which you can activate your core, so you're best off engaging your shoulders to pivot you upwards.

Progression

As I mentioned earlier, you will most likely be starting at the very bottom or close to it, no matter your training experience level. This is perfectly fine. Figure out your level using the method previously mentioned and work your way up.

Flat Knee Raises

Lie down on the floor, bend your knees at 90 degrees and bring them upwards as much as possible. Remember to breathe out on the way up and in on the way down. Keep your spine in as neutral a position as possible. Remember to swivel your pelvis upwards to fully engage your core.

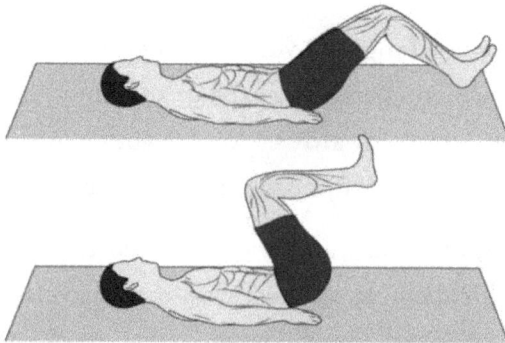

Begin by doing 3 sets of 4 reps (4,4,4). Work your way up to 3 sets of 8 reps to move on to the next progression (8,8,8).

Flat Bent Leg Raises

In this variation, you'll still be lying on the floor, but instead of bending your legs 90 degrees at the knee, you'll be keeping them upright with a slight bend in them. Lower your legs to the floor without touching it and bring them back up. When tilting your pelvis up, don't exaggerate the movement and bring your entire lower back off the floor. Keep it as natural as possible.

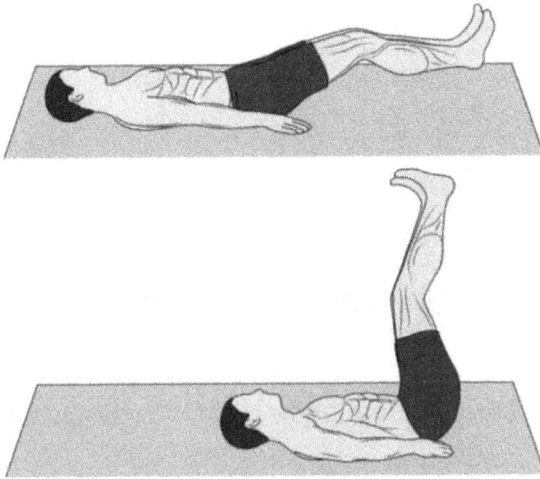

Begin by doing 3 sets of 4 reps (4,4,4). Work your way up to 3 sets of 8 reps to move on to the next progression (8,8,8).

Flat Straight Leg Raises

This variation is the same as the previous exercise except instead of bending your legs when vertical; you'll keep them straight. Remember not to touch the floor on the way down.

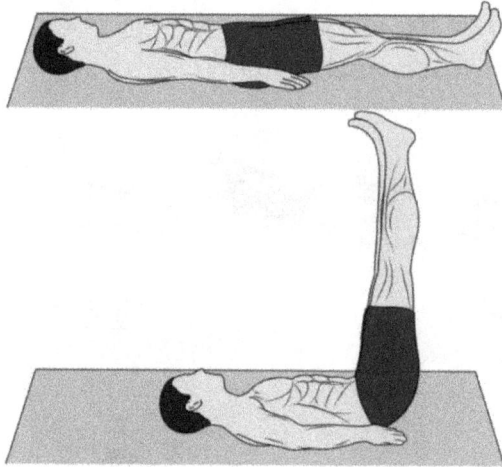

Begin by doing 3 sets of 4 reps (4,4,4). Work your way up to 3 sets of 8 reps to move on to the next progression (8,8,8).

Hanging Knee Raises

While hanging from an overhead bar, which can be the same as your pullup bar, bring your knees up until your thighs are parallel to the floor and gently lower them. You will need to engage and contract your core muscles in order to bring your knees up.

The exact height to which you bring your knees depends on how your body is structured. This is why paying attention to the placement of your thighs is essential. Make sure you keep your arms and shoulders in a neutral position. You don't need to hang limply from the bar, but you shouldn't be pulling yourself up in order to get your knees to rise either

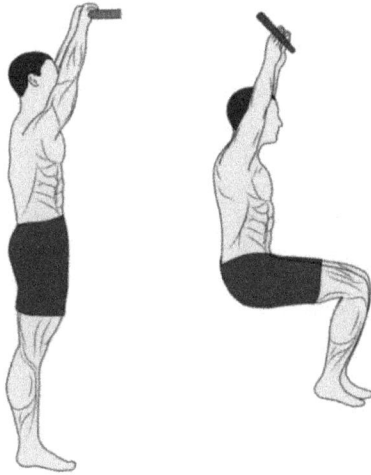

Begin by doing 3 sets of 4 reps (4,4,4). Work your way up to 3 sets of 8 reps to move on to the next progression (8,8,8).

Hanging Bent Leg Raises

This is the same as the hanging knee raise, except you'll be bending your legs slightly while lifting them. Raise them roughly beyond a 90-degree angle and gently lower them. Your legs should be between a knee raises and a straight leg raise. The objective is to raise your knees to a height that is higher than a knee raise (about parallel to the floor) but isn't touching the bar overhead.

Do not raise your legs by activating or engaging your shoulder on the upward motion. Use your core muscles as much as possible to do this.

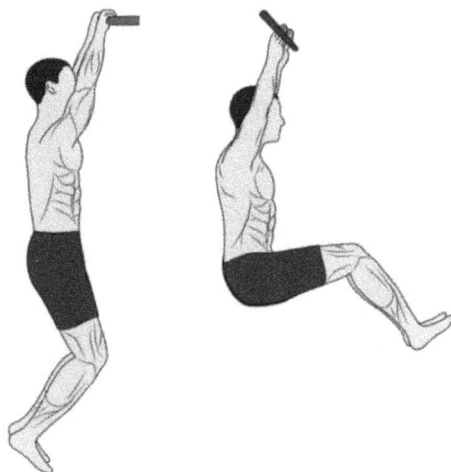

Begin by doing 3 sets of 4 reps (4,4,4). Work your way up to 3 sets of 8 reps to move on to the next progression (8,8,8).

Hanging Straight Leg Raises

Hang yourself from an overhead bar and bring your legs up to a level where they're parallel to the floor. Gently lower them and repeat. Remember not to engage your shoulders to activate the upward movement. You should be activating your core muscles to pull your legs upwards.

You don't need to hang from the bar as a deadweight, either. Support yourself well using your shoulders, but don't engage them or your lats to pull your legs up.

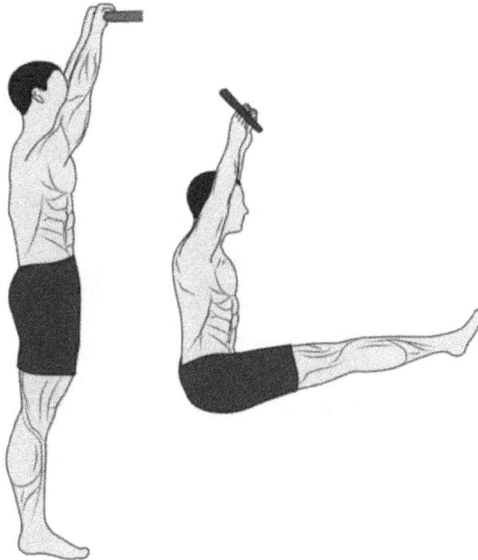

Begin by doing 3 sets of 4 reps (4,4,4). Work your way up to 3 sets of 8 reps to move on to the next progression (8,8,8).

Hanging Bent Leg V-Raises

Bend your legs at a 45-degree angle and bring them up until they're level with your shoulders. Keep your arms as straight as you can throughout the motion. You will need to engage your shoulders to some extent to perform this exercise. You might find the need to swing your legs at the bottom to get some momentum before the upward push, but do not do this.

Remember to reach the bottom in as controlled a manner as possible. Descend too fast, and you'll begin to swing like a pendulum. Lift your legs by contracting your abs and core instead of pulling up with your shoulders and then swiveling your hips upwards.

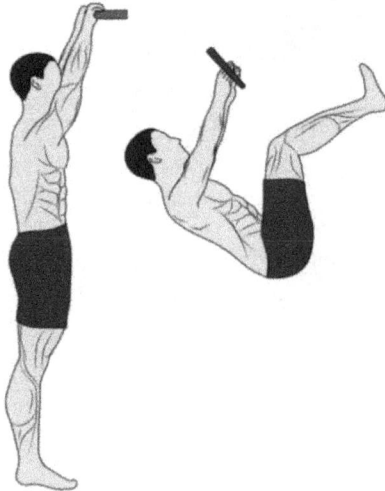

Begin by doing 3 sets of 4 reps (4,4,4). Work your way up to 3 sets of 8 reps to move on to the next progression (8,8,8).

Hanging Straight Leg V-Raises

The same setup as before, but this time instead of bent legs, you'll be keeping your legs straight and touching your toes to the top of the bar. The key here is to make sure you don't use your shoulders too much. You will engage them to the extent that they keep you stable on the bar, but don't contract your lats to pull yourself upwards.

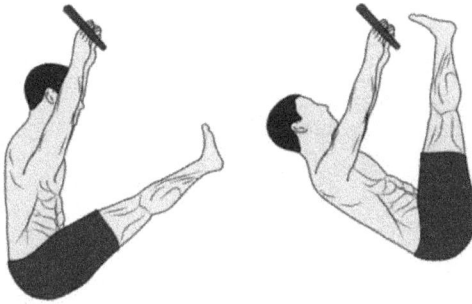

Begin by doing 3 sets of 4 reps (4,4,4). Work your way up to 3 sets of 8 reps to move on to the next progression (8,8,8).

CHAPTER 8:

SUPERIOR SPINE STRENGTH - BRIDGES

The bridge is an exercise you won't find in too many exercise manuals. This particular exercise is borrowed from the world of yoga, where it is commonly called the bridge pose. While yoga doesn't focus on progressions with regards to specific poses, in this chapter, you're going to learn all about them.

Before all of that, though, you might be wondering what's so special about the bridge? After all, if you were to look at a picture of this exercise in action, all you'll see is someone contorting themselves into what looks like an inverted U shape. The efficacy of the bridge goes a lot further than simple flexibility. It is the bedrock upon which the health of your spine is built.

Bridges and You

As I mentioned in the previous chapter, your core consists of muscles in the front and the back. Your back muscles need to remain stable under loading as well as under twisting. Loading refers to when weight or effort is placed on the muscles around the lower back, and it needs to remain stable. As far as twisting goes, it is precisely what it sounds like.

While the spine needs to remain stable, it also needs to be able to move to a healthy degree. Think of the movement as being when you twist your back from side to side. You can train your arms, shoulders, legs, and abs all you want, but these do not directly address the issue of the degree of twist in your spine.

Bridges are what do this for you. In addition to your spine, the bridge also opens up a lot of other joints throughout your body. For starters, it forces your spine to support itself as you raise yourself off the ground. Next, it also opens your shoulder joints and clears and constrictions in the chest and your abs, thereby allowing for a freer flow of air.

In yoga, this is one of the most significant benefits of the pose that is stated. As you can imagine, a great deal of emphasis is placed on yoga about the energy flowing through the body and the free flow of it at all times. While we're not so concerned with this aspect of bridges, there's no denying that you will feel more energized once you execute a bridge.

Despite its somewhat convoluted looking structure, the bridge functions best as a relaxing pose. This is because it opens your joints and extends the front of your body and respiratory system. In addition to this, it also opens your hips and gives you a good stretch, thereby increasing blood flow throughout your body.

Soreness and muscle stiffness usually evaporate once you perform the bridge well. As with all exercises, you need to perform it with good form, or else it isn't of much use. The other benefit of a good bridge is that it will help your performance in other exercises thanks to the overall flexibility it brings about.

All in all, the bridge is an exercise that exposes your weaknesses throughout your body. If there's any joint or muscle that is out of place or sore, you'll immediately feel it. Now, most trainees shy away from this sort of thing because it doesn't bring immediate progress and can be discouraging. However, this is the wrong way of looking at it.

You should welcome exercises such as the bridge because it lets you know exactly what to focus on in your next workout. Therefore, as you read through this chapter, remember that the benefits of the bridge are two-fold. First, you're strengthening your spine, and second, you're getting to know your body better to make it stronger the next time around.

Lastly, performing bridges also leads to a reduction in lower back pain issues since it strengthens your spine. Older people generally benefit greatly from this exercise.

Form

The variation of the bridge I will be referring to here is the full bridge. This is the same as the yoga pose of the same name. You start by lying down on the ground. Bring your arms up and place your palms slightly above your shoulders, with the palms flat on the floor. Thus, your elbows will be bent, and your wrists will be bent in such a way that your fingers will be pointing towards you.

Bring your feet closer by bending your knees. Bring them to a position that is as close to you as possible. Next, drive your body up whatever muscles you can recruit. Use your heels to lift your lower legs off the ground and squeeze your glutes to push your midsection further up.

Push your palms down into the floor and lift your chest as well. Stretch your abs and front core to generate as much of a bend as you can and hold them tight to stabilize yourself once fully off the ground. Believe it or not, this is the easy bit. The tough part is exiting the pose and lowering yourself back down without injuring yourself.

You need to lower both the upper and lower portions of your body simultaneously. Your lower body will want to descend a lot faster, so squeeze your glutes to minimize this. Alternatively, you can focus on lowering your upper body back down to the ground by trying to reconnect your upper back and the back of your shoulders with the ground first.

Following this, you can gently lower your glutes and your thighs back down. When you first perform this exercise, you'll likely find that your glutes fall to the floor with an almighty thud. Squeeze your glutes as much as you can to avoid a freefall situation and perform the exercise on a soft surface to minimize any discomfort.

When in the pose, you can push your abs towards the ceiling to increase the amount by which you'll bend. Don't overdo this too much. The higher you go, the less stable you'll be, so try to find that fine line between challenging yourself and losing stability completely. Remember to keep your heels planted on the floor at all times and don't shift your weight to the toes or lift the toes off the ground completely.

The entirety of your foot should remain planted. Weight distribution is also critical in the bridge. Your wrists will be bearing a lot of the load since your body will automatically push backwards onto them. You can push back using your wrists to drive your weight back down your body.

Progression

Given the complexity of the exercise, there are several progressions to the bridge. Let's look at them one by one. As always, find your ideal level by using the method indicated previously.

Short Bridges

Lie down on your back with your hands by your side. Place your palms down on the floor. Bend your legs at the knee and bring them up to a 45-degree angle. With your feet firmly planted on the floor, squeeze your glutes and raise your torso off the floor. Utilize your leg muscles and rest yourself on your shoulders. Do not put your weight onto your neck.

Gently lower yourself, and don't drop yourself down to the floor.

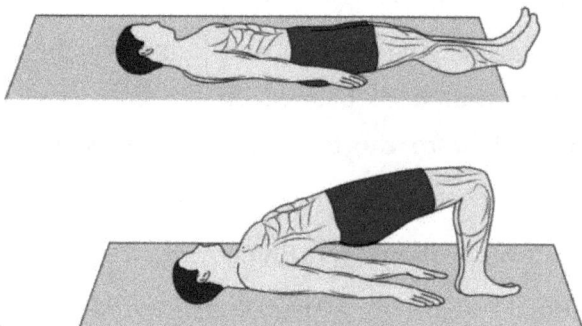

Begin by doing 3 sets of 4 reps (4,4,4). Work your way up to 3 sets of 8 reps to move on to the next progression (8,8,8).

Straight Bridges

Sit on the floor upright with your legs fully stretched out in front of you. Place your arms by your side and contract your glutes and core. Now, lift yourself off the floor using your arms and balance your lower body on the back of your heels. Gently lower yourself to complete one rep.

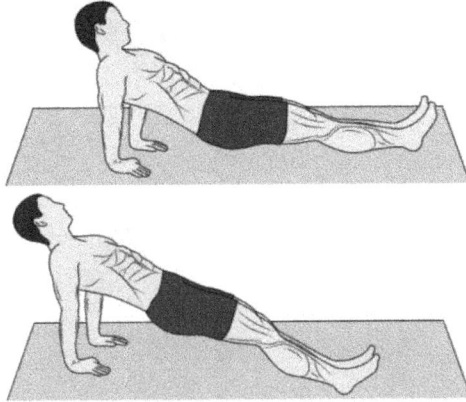

Begin by doing 3 sets of 4 reps (4,4,4). Work your way up to 3 sets of 8 reps to move on to the next progression (8,8,8).

Angled Bridges

This is a tough variation at first, but with practice, you'll get it. You'll need a bench or a small chair for this to work. Stand in front of the platform and bend backward until your body is almost horizontal, and you can support yourself on the chair/platform with your head looking backward(upside down.) Keep your feet firmly planted on the ground.

If you find your toes coming up off the ground, then you're probably leaning too far back. If the extremity of the platform is somewhere near your hip, it's too close, and you should create some distance between it and yourself. Push yourself up with arms extended and lower your self to the starting position.

To exit the pose, lower your hips to the ground gently and sit down on the floor and bring your arms back by your side.

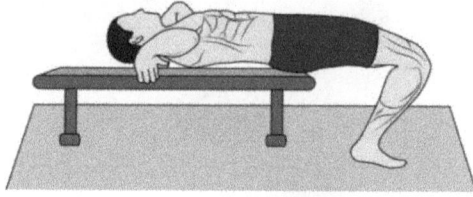

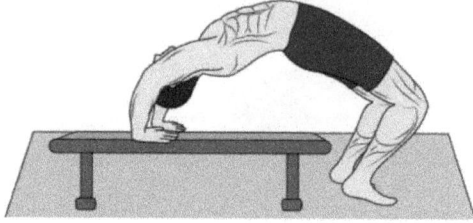

Begin by doing 3 sets of 4 reps (4,4,4). Work your way up to 3 sets of 8 reps to move on to the next progression (8,8,8).

Head Bridges

This exercise is the same as the previous one, except you won't be resting on the platform. Instead, you'll go all the way down and rest your hands on the ground. Hold this position and gently aim to touch your head to the ground.

Hold this position and then lower your back down to the ground gently in order to exit the position.

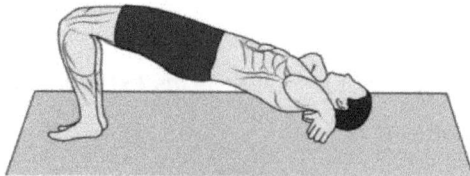

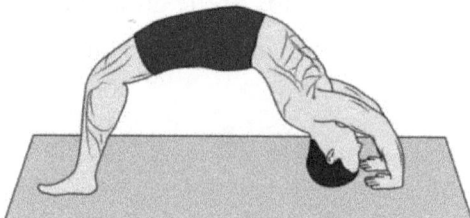

Begin by doing 3 sets of 4 reps (4,4,4). Work your way up to 3 sets of 8 reps to move on to the next progression (8,8,8).

Half Bridges

You will need a circular prop or an exercise ball of some kind for this. Alternatively, you can use a soft prop. Place this under your lower back and lie down with your feet planted firmly on the floor. Now, contract your core muscles and lift your lower back off the prop and support yourself on your hands and the balls of your feet. Gently lower yourself back down and take care not to drop yourself onto the prop.

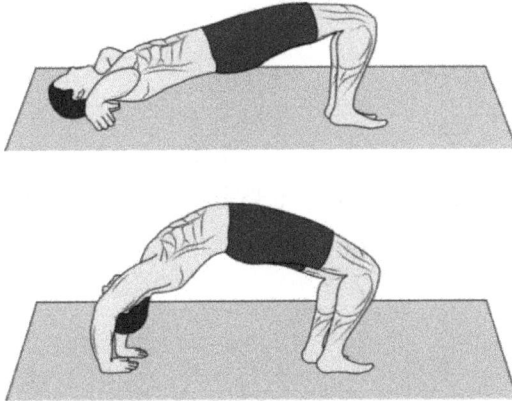

Begin by doing 3 sets of 4 reps (4,4,4). Work your way up to 3 sets of 8 reps to move on to the next progression (8,8,8).

Full Bridges

The technique for this has already been described above. Start by laying on the ground and extending your arms back, with elbows fully bent behind you. Make sure your palms are flat on the floor. Push yourself up off your palms and heels until you form an inverted U position with your body. Hold this position and then gently lower your back down to the ground in order to exit the pose.

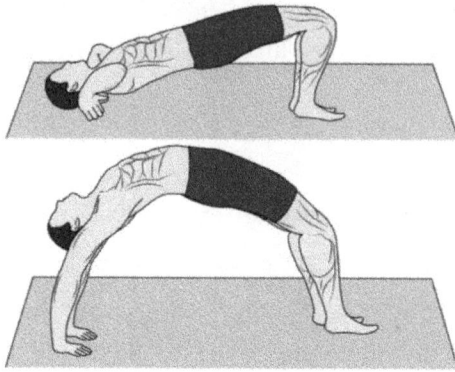

Begin by doing 3 sets of 4 reps (4,4,4). Work your way up to 3 sets of 8 reps to move on to the next progression (8,8,8).

Wall Walking-Down

Stand at a rough distance from a wall from where you can assume a bridge position. Lean backward and place your palms fully on the wall. Now, gently start walking downwards until you reach the bottom into a full bridge pose.

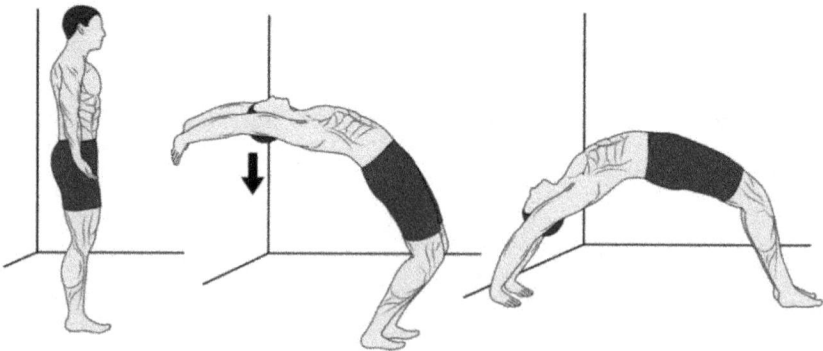

Begin by doing 3 sets of 4 reps (4,4,4). Work your way up to 3 sets of 8 reps to move on to the next progression (8,8,8).

Wall Walking- Up

Complete walking down the wall, but instead of lowering yourself to the ground, hold your position there for a second or two. Now, walk your hands back up the wall gently and work yourself into a standing position. This is a challenging exercise, so take it easy at this point.

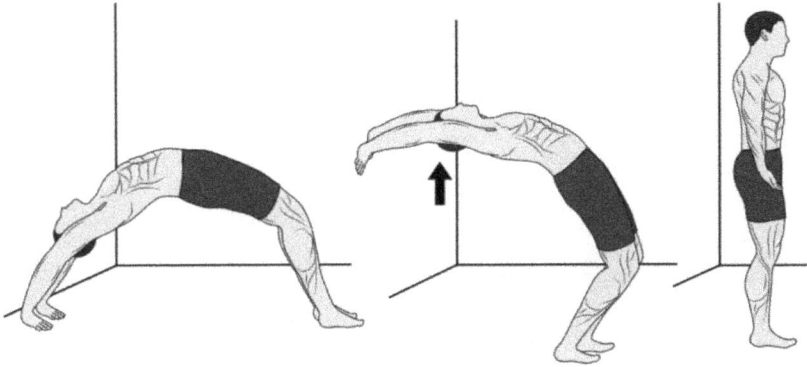

Begin by doing 3 sets of 4 reps (4,4,4). Work your way up to 3 sets of 8 reps to move on to the next progression (8,8,8).

Closing Bridge

At first glance, this exercise will seem impossible. Stand upright and gently begin leaning backwards. You will eventually reach a point where you can no longer maintain balance on your feet. At this point, look backward, upside down, and throw your arms out behind you for support while descending. Lean backwards until you land in the bridge pose. Hold this position. Now relax and start the exercise again from standing.

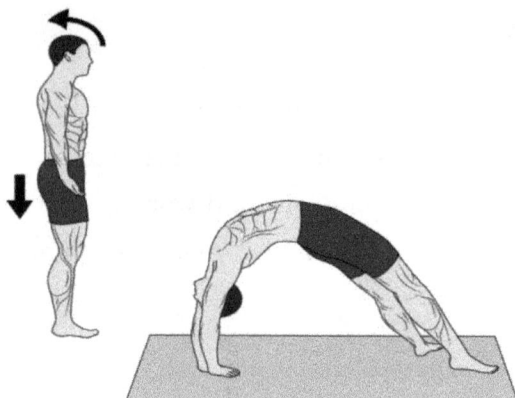

Begin by doing 3 sets of 4 reps (4,4,4). Work your way up to 3 sets of 8 reps to move on to the next progression (8,8,8).

Stand to Stand Bridge

This variation is exactly the same as the previous one, but it requires you to stand back up from the bridge position up to a fully upright position. Flip back into a bridge pose and, as gently as you can, then flip back into a standing posture. This is as hard as exercises get, and you will need almost perfect body control and flexibility to pull this off.

Throughout all the progressions of the bridge, make sure you keep your feet planted on the ground. Don't let your toes rise off the ground, and don't use your heels to solely support yourself.

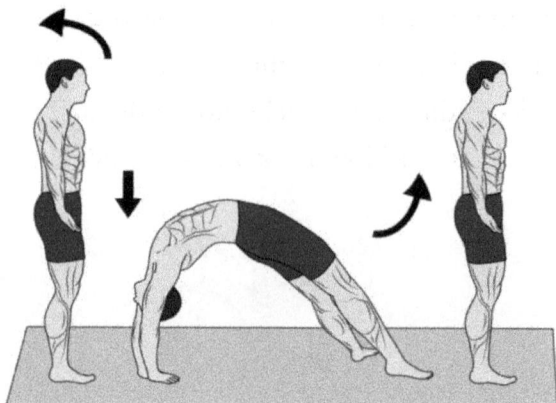

Begin by doing 3 sets of 4 reps (4,4,4). Work your way up to 3 sets of 8 reps to move on to the next progression (8,8,8).

CHAPTER 9:
POWERFUL, HEALTHY SHOULDERS

Your shoulders are the final part of your body we will be targeting in this routine. The importance of healthy shoulders cannot be overstated. Given that your shoulder joint is what connects your arms to your torso, it goes without saying that this joint assumes a lot of work every time you perform any physical activity.

There is an aesthetic part of all of this as well. Healthy shoulders tend to pop and give your body a more rounded look. In men, big shoulders accentuate the V shape of their torso, while healthy shoulders tend to give women a healthier look and dispel any notion of physical weakness.

If you wish to lift anything, including your body weight, it is crucial for you to train your shoulders correctly.

Handstands and Shoulders

Your shoulders can be subdivided into three components, often referred to as heads. While the medical terms for these are different, you can think of them as being the front, middle, and back head. The thing that makes shoulders tricky to train and balance is that even compound movements tend to hit only two heads most of the time.

One of the most common strength training exercises in the gym is the overhead press or simply the press. In this exercise, you stand up tall and lift a weighted barbell over your head and bring it back down close to your chest before lifting it back up again. This exercise doesn't hit the back of the head with too much force, and as a result, you'll find that most gym trainees tend to have underdeveloped back shoulder heads.

The only way to ensure you train all heads evenly is to perform a combination of compound as well as isolation exercises. This means more time spent in the gym and more opportunities to get injured by performing an exercise with poor form. I'm not saying that you should not train in the gym, it's just that if you have the option of performing one exercise that can target your shoulders effectively, why do you need to focus on anything else?

This is where handstands come into play. To be more precise, I'm talking about wall handstand pushups. The name pretty much conveys what the exercise is all about. You'll be upside down, supported against a wall, or slightly away from it, and you'll be pushing yourself up and down.

The reason wall handstand pushups are so effective is due to the fact that they recruit more than just your shoulders in order to deliver strength and stability. Your triceps and arms need to work overtime to stabilize and push you. Your lats need to engage in order to perform an effective handstand pushup.

Most important of all, the three heads of your shoulders need to work together to execute the exercise flawlessly. Your traps will also be bearing significant weight, and this is one of the few exercises that will target them. Aside from the fantastic physical benefits, there's the vanity factor as well.

Simply put, how many people do you know who can execute a wall handstand pushup? Forget a handstand, how many do you know who can execute a regular pushup perfectly? Odds are this number is not going to be very high. Performing a perfect handstand pushup is going to give you serious bragging rights.

All jokes apart, though, handstands simulate the real-life action of lifting something over your head using your body weight and helps you maintain good shoulder health.

Form

The final posture of the handstand pushup is easy enough to understand. You'll be upside down and will support yourself against a wall as you push up and down. To execute this correctly, you'll need to pay special attention to your form to make sure you don't injure yourself. Furthermore, good form ensures that everything stays close to one another, and you won't lose stability.

You first need to ensure your feet are firmly placed against one another. It even helps to tense your leg muscles to make sure they don't start flapping around. This will cause an imbalance, and you're likely to have your feet come crashing down to the ground if you do not keep everything tight.

Your arms need to be straight. Think of them as forming a straight line that runs right into the floor. You'll be supporting yourself on your palms, and your wrists will also be supporting a significant amount of weight. This is where bridges come in handy since they'll help immensely with wrist flexibility.

An excellent way to balance yourself is to spread your fingers as wide as possible on the floor. Make sure that your middle finger is in line with your elbows.

Next up is your head. Most people tend to tense their facial muscles or their necks when performing the handstand pushup. This is not a good thing to do. Instead, maintain as neutral a position as possible and move your head in line with the rest of your body. Think of it as being cemented onto your torso and not as an independent thing.

Lastly, getting your breath right is crucial to performing the handstand pushup correctly. Breathe incorrectly, and you'll lose all sense of stability and strength. The correct way to do this is to inhale as you descend and exhale your breath and tighten everything as you push back up.

Doing this makes sure that you'll have an adequate amount of force on the pushup leg of the exercise, and you won't run out of breath when it's most needed. Throughout the exercise, make sure you tighten your abs and everything else you can think of. Tightening your muscles causes your body to focus more of its strength where it's needed the most, and you won't risk having something fall out of place and destabilize you.

Progression

Handstand pushups seem intimidating, but rest assured that by following these simple progressions, you'll be doing them like an expert in no time. The key is to execute each and every step of the progressions with perfect form and not rush along and try to bite more than you can chew. For all of these progressions, start off with (4,4,4) as explained previously and progress to the next level once you can perform (8,8,8.)

Incline Pike Pushups

These are also called incline military press pushups. You will need a bench or a platform to execute these. Place the platform in front of you and bend down towards it. You want to bend at the waist and maintain your head and torso in a straight line. Lower yourself towards the bench by bending at the elbows and perform a push up.

Lower your head to a point where it is close to your hands. From this position, raise yourself back up again, much like you would in a pushup. Raise yourself back up to your starting position.

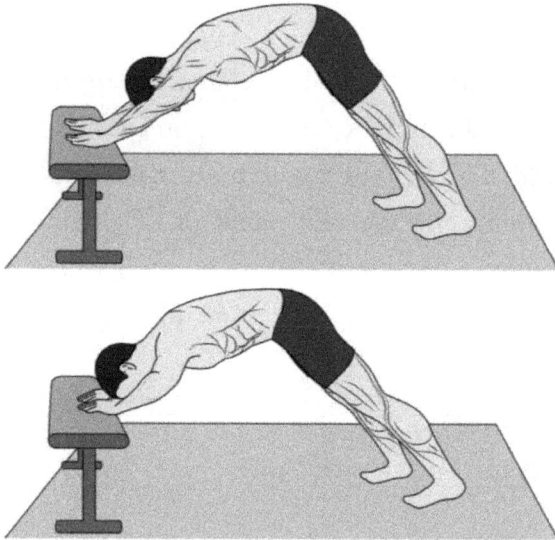

Begin by doing 3 sets of 4 reps (4,4,4). Work your way up to 3 sets of 8 reps to move on to the next progression (8,8,8).

Pike Push Ups

Remove the bench and lower yourself all the way to the floor. Try to keep your feet as planted as possible. Make sure your head travels in a straight line between your arms and keep it in a straight line with your arms and torso.

Once again, make sure your elbows don't flare out to the side and that you breathe in on the way down and exhale as you push yourself back up from the lowest position.

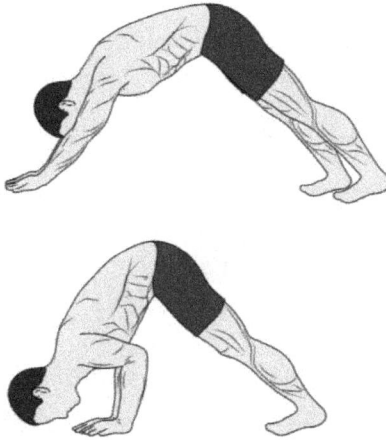

Begin by doing 3 sets of 4 reps (4,4,4). Work your way up to 3 sets of 8 reps to move on to the next progression (8,8,8).

Wall Bent Waist Handstand Diamond Pushup

These are the same as the previous exercise version, except you'll be placing your hands in the diamond position.

Begin by doing 3 sets of 4 reps (4,4,4). Work your way up to 3 sets of 8 reps to move on to the next progression (8,8,8).

Pike Diamond Push Ups

The exact same exercise as above but this time place your hands in the diamond formation, with your thumbs and index fingers touching one another. Lower and raise yourself back to the starting position. Make sure your elbows don't flare outwards and that you exhale on the way up and inhale on the way down.

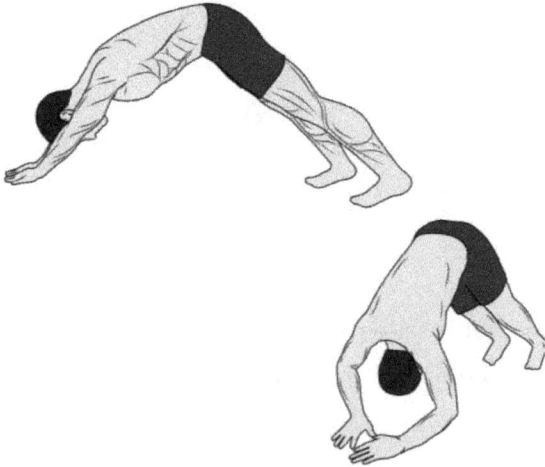

Begin by doing 3 sets of 4 reps (4,4,4). Work your way up to 3 sets of 8 reps to move on to the next progression (8,8,8).

Decline Pike Push Ups

Bring the platform you used in the first variation back, and instead of placing it in front of you, place it behind you instead. Place your feet on top of the bench and lower yourself with your arms out to your side and your head in a straight line between them. Remember that your torso should be perpendicular to the floor and your head in a straight line with it.

Remember to not flare your elbows out to the side and exhale on the way up and inhale on the way down.

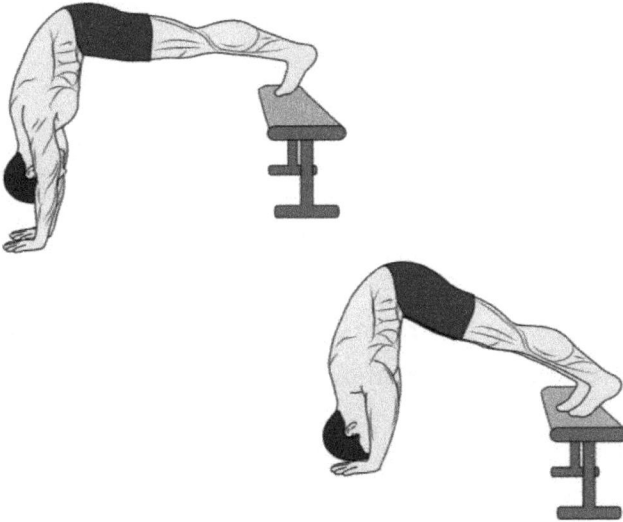

Begin by doing 3 sets of 4 reps (4,4,4). Work your way up to 3 sets of 8 reps to move on to the next progression (8,8,8).

Decline Pike Diamond Push Ups

The same exercise as the previous one, but this time you'll be placing your hands in the diamond formation. Remember to maintain proper form; otherwise, it doesn't count! Keep your elbows tucked in and breathe on the way down and exhale on the way up.

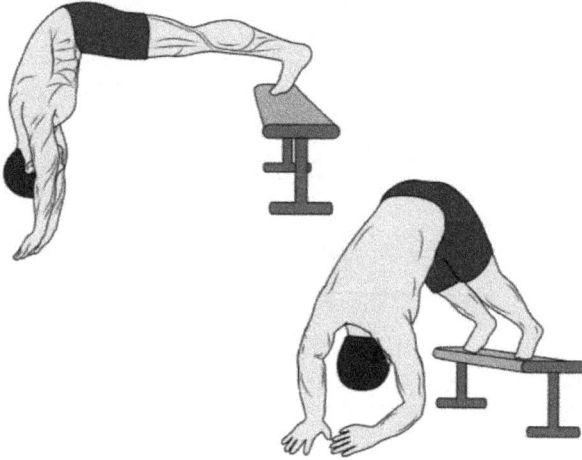

Begin by doing 3 sets of 4 reps (4,4,4). Work your way up to 3 sets of 8 reps to move on to the next progression (8,8,8).

Wall Bent Waist Handstand Pushup

Begin by being in a plank position close to a wall and walk your feet up until you reach a stable point. You don't need to go all the way up. The key is to keep your waist bent. Finding the exact distance you need to be from the wall might be a little tricky, so take your time with this.

Your face will be facing the wall as you lower your torso and head in line with one another and in between your arms. Once you've lowered yourself, raise yourself back up to your starting position, and complete your reps. Walk your legs down the wall back to the ground to complete the exercise.

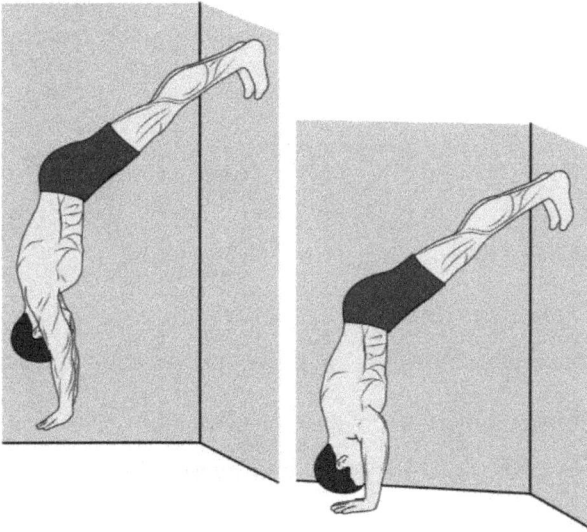

Begin by doing 3 sets of 4 reps (4,4,4). Work your way up to 3 sets of 8 reps to move on to the next progression (8,8,8).

Kick Up to Handstands

This variation requires you to have excellent core stability. Make sure you're in an open space, and there aren't any objects nearby where you could hurt yourself. Position yourself in an inverted V shape on the floor with your palms out in front of you and your legs primed on your toes.

Now, kick up and bring your legs up while simultaneously supporting yourself on your palms. Tighten your core muscles to make sure your legs manage to stay upright and unsupported. Hold this position for 5 seconds at first and work your way up to 20 seconds. This exercise is so you can safely position yourself in the correct handstand position against the wall.

Wall Half Handstand Pushup

As the name suggests, this is a half version of the exercise. Place yourself against a wall, upside down, and lower yourself until your arms are half bent. Push yourself up until your elbows are almost locked. You can place your toes gently along the wall to stabilize yourself easily.

Do note that you will be facing away from the wall when performing this. In other words, your back will be towards the wall.

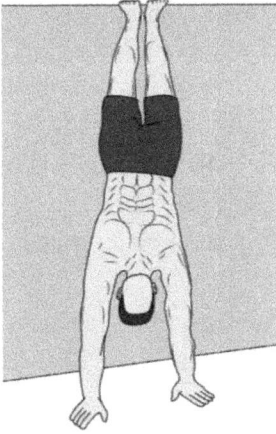

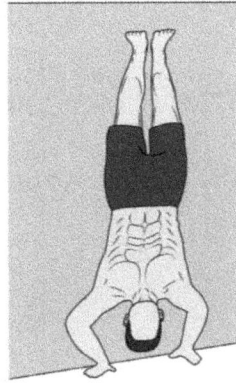

Begin by doing 3 sets of 4 reps (4,4,4). Work your way up to 3 sets of 8 reps to move on to the next progression (8,8,8).

Wall Handstand Pushups

Perform the full exercise as previously detailed, except of going halfway, you will be going all the way down. Make sure your head touches the ground very gently at the bottom. Remember to lower your head to the point where it touches the ground lightly. All the while, maintain a tight core and take note of your stability during the routine. Now push yourself back up to the starting position to complete your reps.

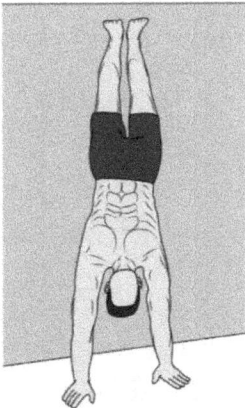

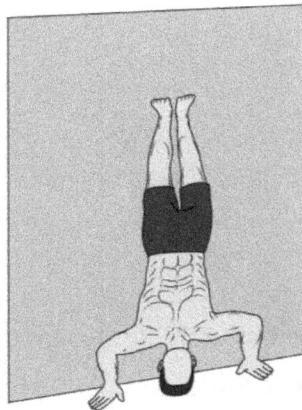

Begin by doing 3 sets of 4 reps (4,4,4). Work your way up to 3 sets of 8 reps to move on to the next progression (8,8,8).

Wall Handstand Diamond Pushups

The same as the previous exercise, but this time place your hands in the diamond shape.

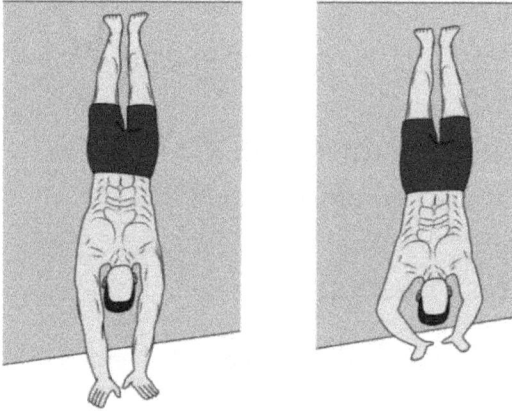

Begin by doing 3 sets of 4 reps (4,4,4). Work your way up to 3 sets of 8 reps to move on to the next progression (8,8,8).

Wall Raised Handstand Pushups

Instead of balancing your hands on the floor, place them on any raised object such as on some paralette bars for the best performance and safety. Perform the exercise as detailed previously. The higher the object is from the floor, the greater is the range of motion you will subject yourself to. Increase this gradually as you build your expertise at this.

Lower yourself as with the handstand pushup described already. You will be sinking lower can perform this exercise near a wall or some other vertical object you can rest your feet on in order to stabilize yourself as you lower yourself once you complete your reps. Then push yourself back up with arms almost locked. Repeat to finish your reps.

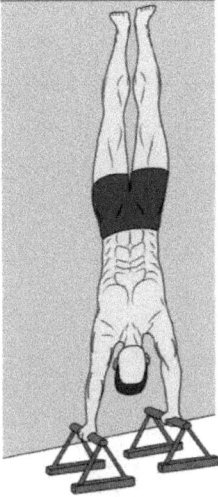

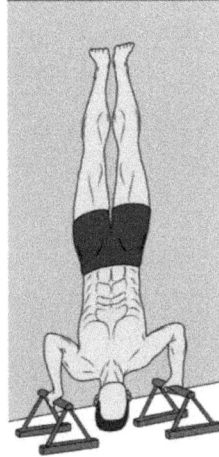

Begin by doing 3 sets of 4 reps (4,4,4). Work your way up to 3 sets of 8 reps to move on to the next progression (8,8,8).

PART 3

BUILDING YOUR PERFECT ROUTINE

CHAPTER 10:
SELF TRAINING

One of the things that will ensure you make constant progress with your workouts is to learn the skill of designing your own training routine and to intuitively understand what works for you and what doesn't. I've mentioned elements of a workout routine throughout this book thus far, but I'll be condensing all of it together in here.

The fact is that once you make progress and develop certain levels of strength, you're likely to find that some exercises work better for you, or some variations feel a lot more comfortable. You might even find that modifying the routine itself works better. Wanting to design your own workout is a perfectly normal thing.

This is why it's essential to understand how you should do this. There are a few elements that go into it. Before all of the technical stuff, it's important to look at the most critical aspect of exercise and workout routines.

Listen

A lot of people skip working out entirely or settle for unchallenging workouts due to the fear of injury. Getting injured and working out is thought to go hand in hand, and this is an extremely unfortunate development. The desire to continually improve and not get injured while doing so seems to be at odds with one another, but the reason for this is that a gross misconception exists.

Here's the thing: your body is constantly communicating with you concerning how it feels and what it's experiencing. You can choose to listen to it or not. Obviously, when you're completing mundane tasks such as brushing your teeth and so on, you don't need massive levels of input from your body. This is not the case when exercising.

One of the things that makes exercise so powerful is that not only does it strengthen you physically, it also develops your mind and body connection. In other words, you'll get to know your body better. More than anything else, this is what prevents injuries. Exercising isn't an activity like playing sports is. What I mean is that when playing sports, there are many external factors that can cause an injury.

Another player could run into you, or you could trip on the ball or whatever object you're handling, and as such, preventing injuries is close to impossible. It usually depends on how lucky you are. In some sports such as football or hockey, it's almost impossible to avoid injuries.

Prevention

When working out, you're exercising by yourself and have complete control over which movements you choose to carry out. The key to exercising well is to find that zone where you're challenging yourself but aren't so far outside your comfort zone where your body just can't handle the movement.

As a beginner finding this zone is a tough task. You've likely never worked out for long enough periods to get to know the signals your body sends you. So what do these signals look like? As with everything else to do with the mind, these signals manifest as feelings. When you try to perform a movement that is well outside your comfort zone, you're going to feel as if it's too tough or that it's uncomfortable.

This is why figuring out your body's signals can be complicated. One of the biggest stumbling blocks in the process is to differentiate between the feeling of laziness and a genuine signal. To be honest, both feel the same for the most part. The difference is in how your body responds to the activity, and you can think of it as a two-step process.

The first step is when you acknowledge the feeling. The second step is you taking action to confirm that feeling. Let's say you're on your way to the gym and feel tired or just don't feel like working out. Your mind is telling you that you'd be better off asleep or bingeing your favorite TV show. Acknowledge the presence of this feeling, but continue doing what you need to do to prepare for your workout.

Once in your workout space, which can be at home or a gym, begin your warmup routine and try to perform the first set of exercises. This is the crucial part. Observe how you feel at this point. Do you still feel tired and unable to complete the workout? Did your warmup leave you even more exhausted or fatigued? Or are you energized and find it easy to continue?

The former is a case of being genuinely tired, and the latter is laziness. Then there's a third confounding case where you'll feel tired but will still be able to perform your workout easily. In such cases, proceed with caution. It might just be that your body is expending a burst of energy to get you through, or it could be a delayed reaction from your mind before it acknowledges that the workout is refreshing. In such situations, it pays to be mindful of your movements and not try to get fancy with things.

If you're pushing for a new level of performance, take it as slowly as you can and ensure you're practicing proper form at all times. Some trainees sacrifice form in order to achieve higher levels of strength. If you're an intermediate level trainee (someone who's been working out for at least three years), then you can safely do this since you'll know when to curb the habit of breaking form.

As a beginner, you should never break form, even if it means you cannot progress. You should never become pedantic about form, but this is something that takes time to develop. What I mean is that if strength gains are your ultimate goal, sometimes you need to make an additional effort to burst past your previous strength levels.

In such cases, you'll find that you won't be able to maintain perfect form. The trouble occurs when you make a habit of this. Intermediate and above trainees understand that breaking form for a rep or two is fine, but if they cannot consistently perform the movement with proper form, then it isn't a real gain.

Signals

Often you will find yourself in the middle of a workout, and your body might send a signal that the upcoming movement is something it cannot do. Again, this is a feeling you'll receive. You might have completed your pushups easily but might suddenly feel that pullups don't sound like a good idea.

It's tough to tell you precisely what you need to do in such situations because so much depends on your intuition. Generally, here's what you can do. Try the absolute minimum you can for a pullup. This means you hang from the bar and try to do a half pullup. Don't rush this and ensure proper form. If you still find it tough to do or if the feeling persists, don't do the exercise.

In such situations, your body has already performed a set of exercises well, and it's unlikely to be a case of laziness. Thus, it's likely that your body is communicating that something is wrong with the muscles that are needed to execute a pullup well. Try the minimum and test this feeling out. Over time, you'll become accustomed to the degree of signals and will be able to determine if you even need to test the signal out.

Generally speaking, you should follow a simple principle when it comes to developing your intuition while working out. To summarize it into a sentence: Always do something. This means that as a beginner, you should pay attention to your feelings and then test them out. Since you aren't experienced enough to figure out what they mean as yet, do whatever you can and see how it feels.

Never go about your workout robotically or treat yourself like one. You're human, and your body will progress at the rate that is best suited for it. If Jane next door is progressing faster than you, so be it. You're perfectly fine wherever you are. Fitness is a very personal thing and isn't something to be compared with one another.

You can compare your strength to commonly accepted standards, but that's where it should stop. Don't look at someone who is at a higher level than you are and wish to be there. Focus on where you're at, and you'll do just fine. Above all else, always listen to your body and develop the mind to body connection.

New Movements

Special mentions must be made about practicing new movements. In such cases, your body and mind aren't used to it, and as a result, they don't know what is going to cause an injury. You will experience discomfort when practicing them, and much like you have to learn to differentiate between laziness and intuition, you'll need to distinguish between the discomfort that comes from unfamiliarity and intuition.

As a rule of thumb, take it slow when it comes to exploring new movements. Practice the form with as low a weight as possible before going all in. Observe your breathing and how your body feels when performing the movement. As I said previously, you want to find that zone where you're pushing your limits but not so far outside it where you'll injure yourself.

Your intuition will let you know where this is, so trust that you'll build it over time. Meanwhile, take it slow and be mindful of the movements you're performing.

Your Routine

The structure of your basic routine has been outlined previously as well as the progression that you will be following. Take the time at this point to review that. You will be performing the appropriate variation of each exercise outlined in this book thus far for appropriate reps, starting with (4,4,4) or (3,3,3) if that variation happens to be too tough. In order to progress to the next level, you will need to perform (8,8,8) or (12,12,12) on certain exercises. Here is what your basic workout routine would look like. Repeat this every other day, or whenever you feel rested enough to adequately perform the workout.

Exercise	Sets/Reps
Dynamic warm up routine	10 min
Appropriate variation for squat progression	3 sets of between 4 and 8 repetitions; Rest between one and 2 min between sets
Appropriate pull up variation	3 sets of between 4 and 8 repetitions;

	Rest between one and 2 min between sets
Appropriate handstand pushup variation	3 sets of between 4 and 8 repetitions; Rest between one and 2 min between sets
Appropriate leg raises variation	3 sets of between 4 and 8 repetitions; Rest between one and 2 min between sets
Appropriate pushup variation	3 sets of between 4 and 8 repetitions; Rest between one and 2 min between sets
Appropriate bridge variation	3 sets of between 4 and 8 repetitions; Rest between one and 2 min between sets
Static stretching routine	10 min

Having said that, if you're an intermediate trainee and are already performing at a high level, you can customize the workout routine to suit your needs better. Generally speaking, rep ranges up to five are suited for strength training programs. Ranges between five to eight are in the realm of strength/hypertrophy.

Hypertrophy refers to a training process that forces muscle fibers to become thicker, and as a result, your muscles increase in size. The strength/hypertrophy rep range ensures that you'll be training for strength as well as size. While you won't be maximizing either one, you'll receive the best of both worlds, so to speak.

Pure hypertrophy reps range between eight to 12. Rep numbers over

15 are geared towards endurance. A thing to note at this point is that as you increase the number of reps you perform, the weight you can lift will also decrease. In order to build muscle, you need to lift as much weight as you can. Training for endurance is not going to build muscle.

This doesn't mean you shouldn't train your cardio system. It's just that your training shouldn't be optimized around it unless you're looking at becoming a professional marathon runner. For everyday purposes, training in the strength/hypertrophy range is ideal.

Rest Periods

The rest periods corresponding to each rep range are different. Strength training routines tend to have more extended rest periods, which can be up to five minutes and start from two to three minutes. Strength/hypertrophy training requires rest between two to three minutes between reps, although you can rest for shorter periods.

Hypertrophy training calls for rest periods of around a minute or so. Endurance training reduces the rest period even less with some programs such as high-intensity interval training having periods of about 15 seconds or so. As you progress, it can be tempting to increase the size of your rest period to enable you to recover better and perform the exercises better.

Understand that the rest periods are a part of the form and are just as important. If you cannot perform the exercise with proper form after resting for the requisite period, then it isn't a true rep.

Splits and Isolation

As I've mentioned earlier, isolation routines (also called splits) are not suitable for a beginner to practice. For intermediate trainers, though, they provide a lot of benefits. The program outlined in this book can be modified to a split program. The advantage of a split routine is that you can target muscles individually, and you can load them up more.

Since you won't be performing as many compound movements, your body will recover faster. Standard split routines call for workouts four days per week or more as compared to three days per week for strength routines. This frequency simply corresponds to how long it takes the body to recover.

Designing a split routine with bodyweight training is a little more complicated since it's not fully possible to isolate your muscles like you can with free weights. As a result, you can follow either a two day or a three day split. You could follow a push/pull two day split, which will have you performing squats, handstands, pushups, and leg raises on the push day.

On the pull day, you can perform pullups, horizontal pulls, and planks, for example. You can add additional exercises if you wish, such as deadlifts and dips as well. I'm not going to go into the intricacies of these other exercises since I'm assuming that as an intermediate trainee, you'll have prior training knowledge of them. Do note that to make a split work well, you will need access to a gym.

A three day split could be on a push, pull, and core and legs and core rotation. An excellent option to turbocharge your splits is to perform supersets. Supersets involve performing two or more exercises in quick succession that target the same muscle. This exhausts the muscle but provides more strength and hypertrophy boosts.

How to Create A Workout Plan

Let state right off the bat that creating a custom workout plan is a time-consuming process. It's easy to write a bunch of exercises down on a piece of paper, but it's entirely another thing to see it through successfully. You'll find that your body will respond differently to each exercise, and rep ranges, as well as volume, so you will need to be adjusting accordingly to how you respond to them.

Designing a great workout routine for yourself begins with your existing training log. Remember how I mentioned that you need to track your progress with your workouts and write down how many reps of each exercise you're performing? Well, this log will form the basis of your own custom-designed program.

Go over the exercises you like performing and make a list of them. Classify them based on push versus pull, as well as the areas of your body they target. Almost every bodyweight exercise is a compound movement, so, for the most part, you will need to ensure there is a balance between the push and pull aspect.

If you find an imbalance between push and pull, you have two choices. You can either find alternative movements to compensate for the ones you don't like, or you can suck it up and do the ones you don't like.

Next, you need to figure out your rep method.

Reps

There are different methods of implementing an exercise rep range. You can do supersets, pyramid style reps, or classic reps. The rep method used in this book is the classic style rep. In this method, the number of reps remains constant, and so does the weight.

Pyramid style reps vary both the weight and the number of reps. Generally speaking, the number of reps is increased or decreased by two. So you could have (8,6,4) or (4,6,8). The weight is accordingly increased or decreased. Cases where the weight is decreased (that is, the reps are increased over sets) are called inverse pyramids. These are considered to be the best when it comes to strength/hypertrophy programs since you'll be lifting the heaviest weight when you're fresh and lighter weight as you become more exhausted.

Designing a pyramid rep range with bodyweight exercises is tough. An option you have is to perform different variations of the exercise for different reps. For example, you could do four diamond pushups, six regular pushups, and eight assisted pushups.

Progress

The next element to figure out is how you'll handle progression and stalling. Stalling can be controlled by dropping down the variation a notch or decreasing the number of reps. Progression is a little more challenging to figure out. You already have a template when it comes to the classic rep range progression in this book.

Pyramids are more difficult to handle. You can choose to add more reps to each set until it hits a specified number. For example, you can start off with (4,6,8) on the pushup progression and increase the number of reps by one every time you workout. Once you reach (6,8,10), you can increase the level of the progression and switch back to a (4,6,8) for this higher level.

In other words, you started off by performing the diamond pushups first. You'll be performing the next, higher progression second and the next progression as your third set. It is a bit more complicated and takes more tracking. The flip side is that you can make better strength gains. As with everything else, there's always a trade-off.

Keep in mind that your workout routine needs to be backed up by good nutritional principles and the right amount of sleep and water consumption. The fanciest workout routine will fail if you don't sleep enough, eat right, or drink too little water.

CONCLUSION

So, are you ready to get fit and strong? Throughout the course of this book, I've tried to convey to you that fitness is a question of applying some basic principles and then backing them up with hard work. It seems intimidating only because of the large quantities of marketing nonsense that exist in this space.

Whether you're a beginner or whether you're over 50 or even 70, getting fit is not a complicated process. Sure, it takes work, but this doesn't mean it's impossible or that you cannot achieve it. It all begins with understanding the basics of exercise and how strength-building works. More importantly, you should understand why you need to prioritize it.

Next comes the understanding of the three fundamental factors that determine your overall fitness: Food, water, and sleep. It seems so simple, but it's often ignored by most people. Ensuring you tick the boxes with regard to all three will do a lot more for your health than any form of exercise you can undertake.

As you do this, you'll need to start working out. This book has given you a great routine to get started with along with giving you directions on how to figure out where you need to begin. Every exercise in this book targets a large group of muscles, and thus your entire body will be receiving a thorough workout.

Remember to perform all the exercises with perfect form since this will prevent injuries and also build actual strength. It will be tempting to take shortcuts, but these won't bring about any real change. Your gains will be temporary and will fade at the slightest hint of stress.

There are many variations to each exercise, so take the time to get to know all of them. Perform them slowly at first, and don't overestimate your abilities. It's better to start slow and achieve steady long term progression than having to stop and start all the time.

Lastly, I'd like to remind you to be patient. You might want immediate gains, but it doesn't work that way. You'll need to be persistent and consistent in your efforts. Before you know it, you'll be there and you will be a different person.

I wish you all the luck in the world. It's an exciting journey you're going to embark on, and it's normal to feel some level of trepidation and nervousness. You may also be feeling some form of excitement! Use this to fuel you further and remember, nothing is impossible!

REFERENCES

Carroll, A. (2015). To Lose Weight, Eating Less Is Far More Important Than Exercising More. Retrieved 5 February 2020, from https://www.nytimes.com/2015/06/16/upshot/to-lose-weight-eating-less-is-far-more-important-than-exercising-more.html

Cross, N. (2018). What Is a Concentric Exercise? | Livestrong.com. Retrieved 5 February 2020, from https://www.livestrong.com/article/428920-what-is-a-concentric-exercise/

Gunnars, K. (2018). How Much Water Should You Drink Per Day?. Retrieved 5 February 2020, from https://www.healthline.com/nutrition/how-much-water-should-you-drink-per-day

Hadim, M. (2012). How to Squat with Proper Form: The Definitive Guide | StrongLifts. Retrieved 5 February 2020, from https://stronglifts.com/squat/

Most Common Weightlifting Injuries and 5 Tips to Avoid Them. (2019). Retrieved 5 February 2020, from https://www.darkironfitness.com/most-common-weightlifting-injuries/

Myers, D. (2016). 19 Reasons Why You Might Want to Stop Buying Supermarket Meat. Retrieved 5 February 2020, from https://www.thedailymeal.com/eat/19-reasons-why-you-might-want-stop-buying-supermarket-meat-0

Roland, J. (2019). Sleep Calculator: How Many Hours and Sleep Cycles Do You Need?. Retrieved 5 February 2020, from https://www.healthline.com/health/sleep/sleep-calculator

Stoppler, M. (2018). Does Stress Make You Fat?. Retrieved 5 February 2020, from https://www.medicinenet.com/does_stress_make_you_fat/ask.htm

Why bodyweight training. (2019). Retrieved 5 February 2020, from http://www.startbodyweight.com/p/why-bodyweight-training.html

Zandonella, C. (2010). Storing food safely in plastic containers. Retrieved 5 February 2020, from https://theecologist.org/2010/jun/24/storing-food-safely-plastic-containers

SHREDDED SECRETS: BUILD MUSCLE, BURN FAT

7 Cutting-Edge Nutrition Secrets You Need Even If You Are Over 50 - The Bodybuilding Diet Plan for Men and Women

REX BONDS

INTRODUCTION

Exercise is one of the best things you can do for your body, but it is often hard to find the right combination to build muscle, burn fat, and maintain a healthy metabolism. If you have never felt as though your diet has been up to snuff with the newest fads, you are hardly alone. Following a regimen becomes more difficult when the sources you find do not tell you what to do after a mere four weeks of scheduled intense insanity. With so many sources telling the public different ways to become a perfectly sculpted human, it is no wonder that so many people get discouraged when trying to start their own weight- loss and muscle-building journeys.

This book, however, gives you the knowledge to lose weight and build muscle for a lifetime. You will learn everything you need to know about how to build a healthy lifestyle instead of a quick get-skinny-quick scheme that falls apart after six weeks. I will help you achieve the body you want in less than a year if you follow all rules and suggestions in this book. It is guaranteed to help you create and maintain the body you want without tearing a hole in your pocketbook.

This book offers nutritional advice to help you maintain a healthy, nutritional diet, designed for both men and women. The three meal plans will aid in cutting fat, building muscle, or maintaining muscle. This book will specifically address nutritional needs for those who are just starting and endurance athletes and strength builders. The dietary needs for each body type are unique, but all can benefit from the nutritional advice in this book. This book is packed with nutritional advice that will explain what foods and ingredients will do for your body, how vitamins and minerals affect the body, and what time is best to eat or drink and why.

It is quite the claim to say that the best of what you will receive from this book is highly profitable to your health, but I've worked with hundreds of people as a trainer. As an avid bodybuilder and personal trainer for years, I have seen what the correct supplements can do for the body when used properly. It is my passion to work with people, both men and women, to make the right life choices and help themselves become the best they can be. There is nothing to stop you from becoming the best you can be, and it is my passion to help you find success in the world of fitness.

Many have trouble determining just what their bodies need. After all, spending your time building the body of which you have always dreamed is easier said than done. However, *Shredded Secrets: Build Muscle, Burn Fat: 7 Cutting-Edge Nutrition Secrets You Need Even if You are Over 50 - The Bodybuilding Diet Plan for Men and Women* is designed with you in mind. That means by adapting the principles in this book to your life will help you develop healthy practices in life that go beyond the capacity of this book.

When you follow what's outlined in this book, you will learn the necessity for protein, finding the best quality, and understanding how it affects your body. You will also see the benefits of a strong foundation which will provide motivation and direction for your healthy lifestyle journey. The goals you make from reading this book will encourage you to see the best in yourself as you see your body undergo healthy change. By reading this book, you will gain a body that adapts to the changes in nutrition by losing weight, building muscle, and maintaining a healthy physique.

Unlike many other books, you will have the benefit of seeing your lifestyle change as you record your healthy journey. This book is designed to give you the tools to create goals that will make you happier with your body over time. Follow the nutritious diet outlined in this book, and you will receive all the vitamins, proteins, fats, and carbs you will need to reach your goals.

This book is based on fact, and I stand by every one of my rules for a healthier lifestyle. Many who have followed my personal training techniques and changed their nutrition have personally thanked me for my help. My trainees have found that their new lifestyle has not only helped them lose weight, but they also see the benefits of becoming more motivated and decisive. The information that I give to all my trainees is found in this book. Their achievements are a testament to the effectiveness of these rules. Anyone can achieve what they and I have. Nutrition does not have to be hard anymore.

I understand the need for help in a world of declining health. It is easy to become sidetracked on the journey and feel as though you cannot make the changes in your life. I see it all the time. However, those that stick with the routines and meal plans have seen results, and I guarantee that you will too. With my help and expertise, you will have the knowledge and know-how to become a powerhouse in your health community. You will be able to take your dreams to the next level and produce a body of which you will be proud. Regardless of your body, skinny or overweight, you will see your body transform into a strong, powerful, chiseled, toned, and athletic body.

So, what is the rush? As Robert Collier said, "Success is the sum of small efforts--repeated day-in and day-out." The habits you gain today will help you become a healthier person throughout the rest of your life. Even if you have not had a health scare and just want to change your body, it is imperative to start a healthy lifestyle today.

After all, every year you add to your lifetime due to healthy living is another year you get to spend with family and friends.

Nutrition can be difficult if you do not know what you are doing, so it is imperative that you start to make your diet bulletproof today. Once you get the hang of creating a healthy lifestyle for yourself, it becomes so much easier to make the right nutrition decisions. Never let poor information about your diet have a major effect on the way you live your life. Get started today.

Shredded Secrets: Build Muscle, Burn Fat: 7 Cutting-Edge Nutrition Secrets You Need Even if You are Over 50 - The Bodybuilding Diet Plan for Men and Women also has been backed up by hundreds of success stories. I have worked with many women and men, helping them improve their lives through consistent work.

Lao Tzu's famous phrase "A journey of a thousand miles begins with a single step" is profound in its simplicity. If you feel overwhelmed by the thought of starting something completely new, just remember that each journey you take starts with that single step. The days turn into weeks, the weeks into months, and eventually you will feel your best after working with *Shredded Secrets: Build Muscle, Burn Fat: 7 Cutting-Edge Nutrition Secrets You Need Even if You are Over 50 - The Bodybuilding Diet Plan for Men and Women* for a year. Persistence is one of the most important traits of developing into who you can be.

Starting with that single step today--taking a walk, eating fruit for dessert, or drinking another glass of water--will start you on your journey to become successful in your weight loss journey.

CHAPTER 1:

EATING FOR ENERGY: HOW WHAT WE CONSUME AFFECTS OUR BODIES

Eating is important. It is one of the most important aspects that determines the health and wellness of everyone on the planet. A healthy diet can increase your chances for a healthier life, just as a poor diet often results in being unhealthy. Eating, therefore, is not just about the joy or misery of putting food into our mouths, but about creating a healthy life for the future.

Vince Gironda, a professional bodybuilder and trainer, once said that gaining muscle is 80% what you eat and 20% how you train. A proper diet plays a pivotal role in determining how well you will gain muscle and maintain, gain, or lose weight. Therefore, it is vital to know how to eat well to provide a platform for natural muscle growth. Eating provides the energy we need for our bodies. The nutrients we consume either add to detract from how the body's processes, and a poor diet can be as detrimental to building muscle as a proper diet can be to gaining it.

Athletes who spend long hours training for events must watch their diets to remain in top shape. Everything from calories to macronutrients are calculated to make sure they can perform at their highest capacities. Since food is fuel, athletes can optimize their performances through eating both the right amounts of food and the correct combination of nutrients for every meal.

Most people starting their journeys to gaining muscle or gaining, losing, or maintaining weight often find nutrition to be one of the most difficult parts to get right. Years of not knowing how to get the correct combination of nutrients certainly does not help the situation. However, finding the right balance of nutrients is the key to any successful diet. Follow the guidelines in this chapter to set the right balance for yourself.

The Advantages of Bodyweight Training

Calories are often viewed as the enemies of any body transformation journey. After all, most diets cut the number of calories consumed by exorbitant amounts, making keeping a successful diet seem difficult if not impossible to maintain. However, calories do not have to be the enemy when changing your body. In fact, a correct diet encourages you to eat more foods that give you strength when working out. The right diet should give you the proper number of calories to consume while not taking the amount to an extreme.

A calorie is a unit of measurement that determines the energy needed to raise the temperature of one gram of water by one degree Celsius. Of course, that makes little sense when calculating energy for our bodies. The term we commonly use when determining energy for the body is kilocalorie, which determines the energy needed to raise the temperature of one kilogram of water by one degree Celsius. The kilocalorie is commonly referred to as a calorie and is labeled on the back of food items.

The body requires heat to maintain its functions. Basic physics dictates that heat is expended when work is performed. All functions in the body require work, which is why the body remains at a normal temperature of 98.6 degrees Fahrenheit. The calories you consume aid in the body's natural functions. So, consuming more calories allows your body to expend more energy and perform more tasks.

Calories make your body exert energy. Consider when you have fasted or gone without food for hours or days. The growl in your stomach tells you that you need to eat food, and you feel weaker the longer you go without food. Of course, in many instances, you do not need to consume food within a matter of minutes to stay alive because you have a backup fat reserve, but the body is used to the energy you consume when you eat consistently. Changing the routine and forcing your body to use backup reserves often causes it to complain. Once you consume food, though, you will notice that your body is suddenly invigorated and ready to perform normal tasks.

Your body requires energy to maintain basic functions. Even when you are sitting still, your body requires energy to breathe, to pump blood, and other necessary bodily functions. The calories you consume allow your body to operate at normal levels. Therefore, the more calories you consume, the more your body can accomplish. If you eat 3,000 calories every day, your body can theoretically work harder than someone who consumes 1,000 calories per day.

To find optimal caloric intake, however, takes careful consideration of body structure and energy expenditure. If you eat too many calories, the extra calories your body would have used for energy converts into storage, causing weight gain. If you eat too few calories, your body tries to compensate for the lack of energy by consuming storage in the body, causing you to lose weight. The key is to find the right caloric intake that will satisfy your goals to lose, gain, or maintain weight and gain muscle.

According to health.gov, Table 1.1 shows the caloric intake for people aged 18 and up.

MALES				FEMALES			
Age	Sedentary	Moderately Active	Active	Age	Sedentary	Moderately Active	Active
18	2,400	2,800	3,200	18	1,800	2,000	2,400
19-20	2,600	2,800	3,000	19-20	2,000	2,200	2,400
21-25	2,400	2,800	3,000	21-25	2,000	2,200	2,400
26-30	2,400	2,800	3,000	26-30	1,800	2,000	2,400
31-35	2,400	2,600	3,000	31-35	1,800	2,000	2,200
36-40	2,400	2,600	2,800	36-40	1,800	2,000	2,200
41-45	2,200	2,600	2,800	41-45	1,800	2,000	2,200
46-50	2,200	2,400	2,800	46-50	1,800	2,000	2,200
51-55	2,200	2,400	2,800	51-55	1,600	1,800	2,200
56-60	2,200	2,400	2,600	56-60	1,600	1,800	2,000
61-65	2,000	2,400	2,600	61-65	1,600	1,800	2,000
66-70	2,000	2,200	2,600	66-70	1,600	1,800	2,000
71-75	2,000	2,200	2,600	71-75	1,600	1,800	2,000
76 +	2,000	2,200	2,400	76 +	1,600	1,800	2,000

Though this list is certainly not set in stone, it does give a rough estimate of the approximate number of calories to consume each day. Keep in mind that the number of calories to consume when you are working out consistently will change according to how long and intense your workout is.

Carbohydrates

Popular diets have made carbohydrates the enemy, but that could not be further from the truth when gaining muscle. They provide the energy stored in the muscles and are necessary for working out. Carbohydrates are responsible for short-term energy and are typically consumed before a workout session because they provide the body with the punch it needs before working out.

Roughly half of your diet should be carbs, and the more carbohydrates you pack into your meal before a workout the better. Not all carbs are made the same, however. Many of today's carbs are heavily processed, removing many of the healthy components necessary for a healthy diet. Processed foods, such as white bread and white rice, have been stripped of healthy minerals, vitamins, and fiber. Healthier versions of these carbs include brown rice, whole wheat breads and pasta, just to name a few. These selections maintain many of original nutrients, making them ideal for consumption.

But how do you tell the difference between good and bad carbs? Carbohydrates that are low in fats are a good place to start. They will provide your body with the most energy without sending most of the nutrients to long-term storage: fat. Bad carbs, on the other hand, often contain simple sugars and lots of fat. Though often hailed as healthy, many breakfast cereals fall into this unfortunate category. They are carbohydrates, but they do not contain the nutrients necessary to maintain healthy energy. Always check the labels of your food to make sure you are getting as many vitamins and minerals as you can.

Eating the best kinds of carbs, such as vegetables, whole grains, fruits and beans, also helps the body to avoid diseases. The vitamins, minerals, and fiber prevent high blood sugar, which often leads to type 2 diabetes and heart disease. Eating the right carbs has also been linked with reproductive health. Aim for six servings of whole grains daily, and reduce your consumption of sugary or simple carbs. Not only will your energy improve when consuming the right carbs, but your overall health will increase.

Always consume carbs before a workout. Workouts that exceed one hour require the body to contain extra energy. Though it is possible for the body to use fat reserves, it is not as efficient as carb usage. Consider packing away a waffle iron. If you use it a lot, it makes little sense to keep it in a storage facility across town. Instead, you will want to have access to it every morning. I am half-kidding. Though accessing fat is not as dramatic as that, it still adheres to the same principle. The energy it takes to burn energy is easier to access when burning carbs.

If you plan to work out for more than 90 minutes, take into consideration the extra energy you will need to expend. For example, if you plan on working out for two hours, consider increasing your carb intake by two times. Drink two glasses of water with electrolytes instead of one, spacing each sip by 15 minute intervals. Experiment to find the right number of carbs for you before each workout to allow you the best chance of maintaining a high level of energy.

Keep in mind that the number of carbs you eat before a workout is highly dependent on how long you plan to work out, how intense the workout is, and how much you weigh. For example, if you weigh 200 pounds, body-weight exercises will be more intense for you than someone who weighs 150 pounds, even if you work out at the same time. Therefore, there is not one right answer to the number of carbs to eat before a workout. Judge how well you perform with what you consume and make a goal to add or detract from that diet based on your results.

Fluids

Water is the best fluid for your body, and it is also the most plentiful substance. You can get water from the tap at a price significantly lower than any expensive drinks. Water also has all the fluid nutrients you need for working out, and it is remarkably underrepresented when discussing proper health. Though many sources say you should drink eight cups each day, they do not emphasize how important it is to maintain a high level of water in your body.

Fluids are responsible for maintaining a healthy body temperature, for example. Though all animals have some sort of method to keep the body cool, humans are unique in their abilities to sweat through the skin. This keeps the body regulated to prevent overheating and to keep organs working properly. Without a way to cool down, humans would have to stay at home in front of an air regulator to keep from dying. When humans sweat, we can lose several liters, depending on the difficulty of the exercise. To keep the body regulated, you must replace that which is lost by constantly drinking water.

Water is the basis for life. You have no doubt heard that you can survive for long periods of time without food, but water is essential to living. This is predominantly true because the vast majority of your composition is water. 60 - 70% of the body runs on water break downs, the simple decomposition of two hydrogen molecules and one oxygen molecule. Water is essential for burning fat and gaining muscle. Water transports essential proteins and amino acids to and from the cell to initiate basic muscular workings. In essence, without water, you would not be able to do the most basic of functions like breathing or maintaining a steady flow of blood throughout the body.

Drinking enough water plays a part in muscle gain. Since cells need water to perform basic functions, the work done requires access to a lot of water. Lack of water often prevents the muscles from growing at their fullest potential. Consider the last time you worked out without as much water as necessary. Likely, you felt your body lag, not putting forth the same effort as normal. The same event happens at the microscopic level, preventing you from performing your best and building muscle efficiently.

Though thirst is often the most common indicator of dehydration, it is not the most effective. In fact, thirst can exhibit itself in many ways that are difficult to interpret, like hunger or little energy. The best way to determine if you are properly hydrated is through your urine. Dark, low-volume urine is an excellent indicator of dehydration, and light, high-volume urine shows that you are drinking enough fluids.

One of the most common reasons for dehydration is forgetfulness. Most dehydrated people simply forget to drink as much as they should throughout the day, which causes problems later. To prevent that, create a timer on your phone or watch that will remind you to drink every two hours. Try to drink at least one cup every time. The more you drink, the better able you are to maintain a healthy workout pattern.

Remember to drink at least 16oz of water two hours before you hit the gym. Water needs time to circulate throughout your body. Continue to sip water or a homemade sports drink (water or diluted green tea, with added Himalayan salt - a tiny bit of sugar if you are exercising) during the two hours before the gym. You will notice an increase in workout capacity when you have enough water in your system.

Be careful with commercial sports drinks. Though the fruity flavor may encourage you to hydrate more consistently, many sports drinks have a lot of sugar, artificial colors and flavors, and are generally not good for you - you'll end up, in the long-term, hindering your efforts to gain muscle.

Sugars are often stored as fats if not used promptly after ingesting them. These empty calories add to the circumference of your weight without helping you lose other fats. You only need water for the first hour of work. Any additional time spent lifting weights may require additional nutrients from a pre-workout mix, but eating right will also provide them.

Other drinks, such as coffee and tea, are common substitutes for water, but they should not be the only type of alternative hydration you consume. Remember, water is always the best choice for hydration. Limit the number of calories consumed in fluids by not drinking your calories. All alternative liquids should be consumed in moderation.

Vitamins and Minerals

Though you should be able to get all the vitamins and minerals you need from a healthy diet, it is not unusual for some to fall between the cracks. Nutritional eating has become less easy to achieve, especially with fast food chains around every corner, and factory farming methods using depleted soils. However, to gain muscle, you must adhere to a diet that includes these vitamins and minerals.

So, what are the most important vitamins and minerals to add to your diet? Women need more iron until they enter menopause, as they typically lose more iron over the course of a month. Calcium is necessary to keep bones strong. Magnesium is a common mineral to add to the diet to maintain a healthy sleeping schedule. Here are the ten most important vitamins and minerals to consume when building muscle.

Calcium: Calcium is important to strengthening bones, especially for people over 30 years old. As the body passes its peak bone growth at age 30, bones are broken down much faster than they are grown. Osteoporosis becomes vastly more probably if you do not take care of your bones. To prevent bone disease, both men and women should increase exercise time and calcium intake.

Calcium is also responsible for muscles to perform at their best. Calcium aids in transmitting nerve impulses to muscles, which forces them to contract and expand. More than that, however, is the energy that the muscles get when the two types of protein found in muscle, myosin and actin, rub together. ATP keeps your muscles active as you continue to exercise.

Magnesium: Magnesium is one of the most common minerals in your body, but it is also a common mineral to miss. Many people have a magnesium deficiency because it is not as emphasized as other minerals. Magnesium is responsible for keeping the effects of calcium at bay. Calcium builds muscle and causes inflammation, while magnesium reduces inflammation and helps to repair muscle.

Studies have shown that magnesium is responsible for building muscle, repairing the body at an extraordinary rate. Excess amounts of magnesium causes muscles torn from exercise to repair at a faster rate, allowing you to work out more. Magnesium is also responsible for reducing soreness, giving you a more comfortable workout.

Iron: Iron is located in your body in trace amounts. That means that Magneto cannot pull you to the surface of a cell by summoning the iron in your body. However, it is important to keep iron levels up in the body to maintain a rigorous workout session and a healthy recovery. Iron is responsible for moving oxygen to the muscles and transforming carbs into usable energy. Oxygen is responsible for energy transformation and recovery in the body. It is transmitted through red blood cells that send it to other parts of the body.

Since sweat contains small amounts of iron, it is important to keep your levels up. Iron deficiency in athletes prevents them from competing to their fullest abilities. Women are more prone to iron deficiency because of menstruation every month, so it is often necessary for them to take supplements.

Vitamin D: Vitamin D is often known as the supplement that comes from the sun through UV rays. Vitamin D is often referred to as a Rickets deterrent, but that is only one aspect of its benefits: it is also responsible for proper bone and muscle growth. Vitamin D produces hormones that are essential to the body. Testosterone, for example, is often produced as a result of proper vitamin D intake.

The most obvious way to get vitamin D is to go out in the sunlight. However, many overcast areas make that goal less achievable for many. Instead, take a supplement or find it in foods such as fish, dairy, and eggs, though these contain low levels.

Vitamin B12: B12 is a vitamin that is often considered juste one part of a set of B vitamins, which are important to a healthy diet. However, B12 is unique in its part in creating red blood cells. Iron, as mentioned previously, is responsible for using red blood cells to transmit oxygen to the muscles, which makes the pair inseparable.

Vitamin B12 is also responsible for metabolizing fats and proteins. The metabolism drives fat burning and weight loss. B12 aids in breaking down those stored fats and using them in basic cellular activity.

Protein

While carbs determine the amount of energy produced, protein holds the power of promoting quick muscle healing and repair. Proteins are composed of strings of amino acids, which compose muscles and ligaments. Consuming proteins allows your body to adapt to strenuous work, and the additional nutrients will make muscle growth more achievable.

Protein often reduces food cravings when eating correctly. Most people eat too much protein, which is converted to fat. However, eating the right amount of protein can help you lose weight. Also, eating the right kinds of protein can build bone mass. Osteoporosis is often associated with a lack of vitamins in the system, but proteins can aid in preventing it as well.

One of the most commonly referred advantages of protein is the ability for promoting healing. When muscles work strenuously, they create microtears due to heavy exertion. This is manifested in the form of soreness and tiredness. Additional proteins in your diet help to heal those small tears and cause them to build stronger than before. Of course, many consume enough proteins to adequately repair microtears, but adding some to your diet often allows faster healing.

Though proteins are all the rage now, it is a myth that protein is the primary source for muscle growth. Muscles grow through tears and repair. Many who believe this myth, however, often fall into habits of consuming too much protein to their diets. Athletes only need a small addition of protein to their diets to promote muscle growth.

Those who consume much more protein than their counterparts often experience dehydration, increased storage of body fat, undue pressure on the kidneys, and loss of calcium. Eating two meals that contain large quantities of protein is damaging to your health and will prevent you from gaining muscle naturally.

It is another common myth that you must eat red meat to get the most protein. In fact, half of your diet should include proteins from plants. To many, it is difficult to consume beans, vegetables, and legumes on a regular basis, so the rest of the protein should come from lean meat such as fish and poultry.

Tuning to Your Body

Your dietary nutrition is highly dependent on your body. Exercise is recommended for everyone, but some put more into exercise than others. If you find your body lacking strength or energy, adjust your nutrition accordingly. Since everyone has a different shape and size of body, you may need to invest several weeks into finding the right balance for your life.

Keep a journal of your food to monitor how you feel every day when you try new supplements and adjust your diet. If you experience sickness when fine-tuning your diet, consult a physician. This book holds the keys to helping you gain muscle and become more fit, but nothing replaces the professional opinion of a doctor.

CHAPTER 2:
HOW DO MUSCLES GROW? THE SCIENCE OF MUSCLE GROWTH

You may see people at the gym that seem to have all the muscles, that work out constantly, and spend a lot of time in front of the mirror. However, these people may not be as strong as you think. People who are much smaller or hide their muscles behind less definition can often lift more than those with "show muscles." Strength training, after all, is not about simply lifting weights, but how your muscles respond to stimulus from the brain. Gaining muscle does not solely rely on performing any exercise.

Growing muscles often seems much harder than it actually is. In fact, if you use the right tools and follow the right diet, you will see results quickly. However, there is more to growing muscle than visiting the gym. Learning how muscles grow can change the way you work out, ultimately improving your results.

The Physiology of Muscle Growth

Muscles are often damaged while working out. The soreness you feel the day after a hard workout is proof enough of that. The right kind of muscle damage, though, promotes strength and muscle growth. The microtears that occur when a muscle is exercised beyond its capacity forces the body to knit itself back together stronger than before. Protein strands, also called myofibrils, strengthen the muscle fibers forming larger strands visible as muscle growth, called hypertrophy.

Muscles are just like memories: if you do not use them, they will fade. The key to gaining muscle is to make sure you are increasing the number and thickness of muscle fibers faster than they are disintegrating. As the body ages, muscles break down at higher rates, which is why it seemed easier to gain muscle when you were younger. Many believe that if they spend multiple hours at the gym, they will gain the muscle they want, but the key to prime muscle growth is in the down period.

If you do not allow your muscles to heal, they will not grow. It might seem as though you are doing nothing in your down time, but rest is the part of muscle growth that gets the work done. Consider, for example, trying to work on only a few hours of sleep. Though you can still get the work done, you are not retaining as much information nor are you receiving the energy needed to do your job. Muscles need rest to rejuvenate energy sources to give you a proper boost next time you are at the gym.

During rest, satellite cells become more available to your muscles, promoting healthy growth by creating more nuclei to muscle cells. They provide relief to the body on small and large scales and are primarily beneficial in healing injuries. The activation of these cells determines how much muscle is gained after microtears are formed. The debate regarding whether gaining muscle is more natural for some than others is likely linked to satellite cell activation.

The 3 Muscle Growth Mechanisms

Muscles grow because of stressors and changes of pace. This should be obvious when you go to the gym and you feel your body struggle to maintain an excessive load or long periods of stress. The phrase "No pain, no gain" is common among those who work out because it symbolizes what they are doing to their body: as they experience more stress, muscles grow.

There are three main muscle growth mechanisms that ensure muscle growth. Perhaps not surprisingly, they are all affected by how you work out. Runners who compete in marathons tend to have leaner muscles than those who spend hours lifting weights. This is because the types of muscle growth vary per person and exercise. Some are more prone to gain muscle quickly while others are leaner but produce the same results. It all depends on how the body responds to stimulus.

Muscle Tension

One way the many gain muscle is through muscle tension, and it is one of the most common methods. Muscle tension refers to the controlled contracting and expanding of muscles. To gain muscle, fitness fanatics continually add weight to their workouts. If they stay at a consistent rate, they will not see growth. Their muscles will adapt to the pressure put on them and remain in a static state.

Muscle chemistry changes when exposed to long bouts of muscle tension exercises. Satellite cells become active, making it easier for them to repair damage to tissue during times of rest. The motion of moving muscles also affects the way the body builds muscle. Motion is associated with motor control in the brain, and it can create connections with muscle cells.

Muscle Damage

As mentioned previously, muscle damage is the key reason for muscle growth. After all, the body requires something to repair to build it stronger. The body compensates for the lack of muscular strength by healing the muscle fibers in thicker strands.

Muscles are also highly affected by the rate at which they heal. If you are new to exercising, you will no doubt feel the strain of soreness after even one session. After that, however, it may become more difficult to detect when your muscles are changing. Do not be fooled by the lack of soreness after a workout. Satellite cells are activated after difficult workouts, and your body will likely adapt to the changes. It is still vital to rest after working out, despite your level of comfort.

Metabolic Stress

Do you remember the last time you were on the road, running for as long as possible, and you felt as though your lungs were going to burst, your legs were going to give way, and your heart was going to pop out of your chest? Metabolic stress refers to the stress of vital chemical reactions within your body. When you were running as fast or long as you could, you were testing the bounds of your metabolism.

Metabolic stress is one of the most common ways to build muscle because it relies on your body's ability to adapt to change. When you work out, your body can only handle so much stress at one time. However, as you build muscle and your body adapts to the changes in your form, you will notice that working out at that same level becomes easier.

Muscle cells often increase without changing the weight applied. Bodybuilders who focus on the increase in muscle size instead of strength often move quickly from one machine to the next. Glycogen in the muscles force the muscles to expand, making them larger without affecting overall strength.

Hormones and Muscle Growth

Hormones are largely responsible for muscle growth, and the most commonly noted are testosterone, insulin-like growth hormone, insulin, and growth hormone. Each facilitates the growth of muscles through natural processes. Other hormones, such as epinephrine and norepinephrine, also aid in repairing damage.

Contrary to popular belief, testosterone is not solely a male hormone, though men do produce it at a higher rate than women. Testosterone is vitally important to building muscles because it promotes repair work and stimulates growth. Those who exercise experience an exponential raise in testosterone, promoting cells to increase their growth and making them more sensitive to the hormone in the future (Leyva, 2020).

Insulin also repairs damage to muscle by breaking down fats, vitamins, and minerals into usable energy. Those who suffer from advanced type 2 diabetes, or type 1 diabetes need a constant supply of insulin to nudge the hormone into breaking down foods. Proper diet and exercise help produce insulin.

Why Muscles Need Rest

It has already been established that muscles require rest to repair themselves, but what you do during that rest period is also a factor in how much growth you will experience. A proper diet is key to muscle growth. Without it and care for muscles during the growth period, you could cause more harm than good. Though differences in growth also depend on sex, age, and genetics, it could take 24 - 48 hours for the muscles to heal completely.

The Myth of Rapid Growth

Movies showing the rapid growth of muscles are often misguided. Muscle growth is not only hard work, but it also takes time. Under extreme conditions, you may see celebrities boasting of working out several days each week and several hours every day, but healthy muscle growth is not that fast.

If you do not see muscle growth in the first week, month, or even few months, do not be discouraged. Every body has a different composition, and building muscle is easier for some than others. For example, men are more likely to see faster muscle growth than women. Since testosterone is a key hormone in muscle growth, it only makes sense that men, who produce the hormone in greater quantities, experience greater growth. Genetics also play a factor in muscle growth.

However, there are ways to increase the likelihood of faster muscle growth. Making sure your nutritional needs are met is the first step to building muscle. If you cannot get all the nutrients you need from food, use supplements to offset the imbalance. Maintain a consistent exercise routine, and you will start seeing growth faster.

Other Muscle Growth Factors

Building muscle is a highly personal journey. There are other factors that prevent your body from reaching its fullest potential in the fastest way possible. Many of these other growth factors have nothing to do with your diet or exercise routine and are simply a part of your genetic makeup.

Genetics

People who say they cannot build muscle because of their genetic makeup might be right. Though it is not true that you are destined for an eternity of small muscles if you do not have the right genes, there are other factors at play. Everyone has two types of muscles: slow- twitch and fast-twitch. Some, however, have more of one type than the other. Slow-twitch muscles are endurance muscles that do not wear out easily, and fast-twitch muscles contain powerful bursts of energy. If you feel more at home running long distances, most of your muscle mass is slow-twitch. If you find short bursts of energy like sprinting short distances, your muscle mass primarily consists of fast- twitch muscles.

Body type is also responsible for seeing muscle growth. Both endomorphs (people who are built with a round shape) and ectomorphs (people who are built with a linear shape) gain muscle. Endomorphs, however, require more fat loss to show muscle, while ectomorphs show muscle more obviously. Your body type does not hinder you from gaining muscle, but it might prevent you from seeing it.

Age

It is no secret that people under the age of 30 seem to have more luck building muscle than someone in their 60s. Muscle starts to deteriorate at a rate of 1% every year from the age of 50 onward if you do not exercise regularly. So, if you feel like your muscle mass is not the same as when you were in your 20s, you are right.

That does not mean that gaining muscle after 50 is impossible, however. With constant muscle training, you can turn this deterioration around and maintain a healthy amount of muscle throughout the rest of your life. Do not become discouraged if your muscles are not what they used to be.

Training Experience

Having a background in muscle training helps you develop muscles with more efficiency than someone who has never started. After all, someone who has dedicated many thousands of hours to exercising will naturally reap the benefits. Putting in more hours at the gym also means more rewards and greater ability to gain muscle.

Hormones

People who naturally produce more muscle-building hormones will generally see more muscle growth than those who are less fortunate. When the brain does not produce enough chemicals into the body, gaining muscle can be difficult both physically and mentally. Steroids are often seen as an alternative to healthy muscle growth, but they are never the answer. Steroids stimulate growth hormones and are illegal in many events because participants have not achieved their bodies naturally and have growth unnatural for the human body.

Nutrition

If you spend all of your money on fast food, you are not going to see results nearly as quickly as you would like. Nutrition is important to keep your body active, and the food you consume should reflect that. Eating and drinking the right things and in the right quantities can account for 50% of muscle growth (The Mecca Gym, 2017). If you are not gaining muscle through exercise, there is something wrong with your diet.

To gain muscle, add plenty of protein to your diet. Protein is responsible for muscle growth and repair, which aids in keeping your body fit while at the gym and creating the perfect muscle structure once resting. If you plan on gaining serious muscle, consider eating your gram-equivalent weight in protein. Consume one gram of protein for every pound you weigh. Of course, do not ingest more protein than you can burn, or the rest will turn to fat.

While you are increasing your protein, also increase your overall caloric load. However, instead of reaching for an ice cream scoop, use the additional calories to pack your body with energy. Research how much you should consume for both your body and exercise equivalent. Add extra vegetables, fruits, and proteins to your diet to maintain a healthy physique.

Know what carbs you are adding to your diet. Though it might be tempting to grab a bucket of fries and use that as an excuse for your "healthy" carb load, the wrong types of carbs can damage the effectiveness of your workout. Look for carbs that contain a high fiber ratio, preferably 5:1. The more fiber you put in your diet, the more likely you are to see positive results. The wrong types of carbs also increase blood sugar and make you hungry faster. Vegetables are good choices for carbs because they fill your stomach and your energy reserves.

Fill your foods with the right amino acids. Amino acids make up proteins, which are essential in building muscle (as we've discussed), but not all of them are naturally produced in the body. 15 of the 23 amino acids required for protein building are not found in the body and must be consumed. When you do not receive all the amino acids required, your muscles start to break down. Animal products are the most common sources of amino acids. Milk, meat, and seafood all contain the necessary additional amino acids. Though some are found in plants, some are not. Vegans must often use supplements to build muscle at the same rate as those who eat animal products.

Women and Muscle Growth

Women often feel like they are at a disadvantage when it comes to muscle growth. After all, the men who hit the gym seem to gain more muscle quicker than females, much of which has to do with their natural output of testosterone. It is more common to see a highly muscular man than a woman. However, that does not mean that women do not build muscle at the same rate as men. Women tend to focus less on building large muscle mass than men. They often spend more time lowering body fat than gaining muscle. But, through progressive weight increase, they will see the same results as men, so there is no excuse for not building muscle.

Women generally start with a lower muscle concentration than men, so it appears as though they are not gaining muscle as quickly. Women also tend to worry about becoming too bulky, so they stop increasing weight after muscles start to grow at a faster rate.

Testosterone is produced in both men and women, but men produce it as much as five times the rate as women, spurring the myth that men gain muscle quicker than women. However, women produce more IGF-1 than men, a hormone that is also responsible for muscle growth. IGF-1 is responsible for the growth in children, and hormonal treatments often cause muscle growth. The evidence insists that women are just as capable as men in muscle growth.

A lot of muscle building is also in the mind. A study of men and steroids determined that the mind is responsible for creating a boundary for muscle growth. As the saying goes, if you believe you can, you are right, and if you believe you cannot, you are right. A group of men were told that they would receive steroids for a study to determine the effects of muscle growth. One group received hormones and the other a placebo. Far from having no effect, the placebo actually encouraged the bodybuilders to pack on more muscle, approximately 350% more than before, all from the power of suggestion (Shapiro, n.d.). The mind controls the functionality of the body by telling you when to quit. Often, your mind is the first to yield.

CHAPTER 3:

FUELING YOUR TRAINING: NUTRIENT TIMING FOR BETTER RESULTS

Eating is one of the most important parts of muscle growth, as I've stated before. However, there is more to nutrition than simply eating the right things. A vast majority of diets say when to eat certain foods and when to fast. You might also notice the changes in your body fat and energy levels when you eat during different parts of the day. All the changes and energy spikes you feel in your body are due to nutrient timing.

What is Nutrient Timing?

Have you noticed that if you have just carbs for breakfast, you feel less full by the time lunch comes around? Or maybe you have just eaten a late dinner, and the next morning you feel bloated. Situations like these determine how well your body will perform throughout the day. Eating the right macronutrients at the right times not only gives your body energy, it also prepares your body for building muscle.

Nutrient timing makes the most out of your diet by giving you the nutrients you need when you need them. For example, consuming carbs before a workout will give you the energy to complete the task and use energy that has been stored in the muscles. Consuming protein after a workout helps your muscles heal after a difficult workout.

Nutrient timing is the process of setting a schedule for yourself. Not only will you receive the right number of nutrients at the right time, but you will also be able to track what macronutrients are added to your diet. Simply planning when to have which nutrients allows you to see where your diet is lacking and to make up the difference.

Digestion is the process in which your body takes in nutrients and disperses them through your system. Proteins, carbs, fats, and liquids, are all consumed at different rates. For example, fluids and carbs are easily absorbed and likewise easily distributed in the body. Proteins and fats, on the other hand, take longer to absorb into the body. The way these macronutrients digest ultimately determines when you should eat them.

Many advocate for eating carbs before working out and eating protein immediately after, but others believe that protein gives your body that extra boost before a workout. Though there is no exact formula for what to eat and when, review the way your body feels before and after each workout. Everyone has different nutritional needs, so what is right for you may not be right for someone else. Your body composition plays a large role in determining the right nutrient timing. Your body is composed of muscle and fat, and losing more fat than gaining muscle can lead to dangerous consequences. Strike a balance between the two by not starving yourself, but losing fat at the same rate at which you gain muscle.

Why Nutrient Timing is So Important

While it is wise to consider nutrient timing for your everyday diet to make sure you have enough energy throughout the day, it becomes much more important when you eat to gain muscle. Muscle builders require more protein than people who lead mostly sedentary lifestyles, for example. Fitness geeks eat their energy effectively. Carb loading the night before a run is how many endurance racers prepare the night before. The energy located in the muscles makes it possible for them to race faster and endure punishing hours.

Many athletes, however, take an all-or-nothing approach to nutrient timing. If something is "good," they think they should consume as much of it as possible. If something is "bad," they avoid it at all costs (Berardi, 2019). For example, when it was determined that protein would help build muscle and aid in muscle repair, bodybuilders started eating twice what they needed. When sugar was condemned by nutritionists, it received a wide berth, and many bodybuilders refused to add any to their diets.

However, taking this approach often leads to negative nutritional habits. Labeling your food only as "good" or "bad" means you will miss out on some nutritional value that is prevalent in many foods. For example, believing that adding butter to your diet will not aid your journey to building muscle negates its benefits of keeping you full, preventing you from eating processed foods.

To understand how to make the most out of nutrient timing, however, we return to rest days. Your down time determines how quickly your muscles heal and how much energy you have for your next workout. Think of muscle gain as like training a pet. What you do not add to the training, you take away. Giving your muscles the ultimate boost involves eating the correct foods and proportions at the right times. Though you can allow yourself a cheat day every once in a while, the rest of the food you consume should be committed to muscle growth.

This is also true for the other end of the spectrum. Many believe that their off day should deprive them of calories, but these days are the most important to eat the right foods. If you deprive your body of nutrients by cutting too many calories, your muscles will not grow effectively. Many so-called diets often perpetuate the fallacy that eating more on your off days will result in gaining fat, but that is only true if you are not taking care to evaluate the nutrients you eat. Often, you may eat as much as you would on a workout day.

You might notice that on workout day, you do not feel the same amount of energy you do during rest days. When you are satisfied with how much you have eaten after a long day of tiredness, imagine how much your muscles are grateful for the extra fuel to begin their repair.

The body is better able to handle consuming macronutrients by timing the effects each workout has on your body. For example, carbs are more easily digested before and after a workout. The body is more willing to accept carbs after it has been exposed to strenuous exercise. The lump you feel in the pit of your stomach after eating a large load of carbs is often the result of eating too much while sedentary.

It is common to eat foods such as potatoes and yams during down days, but these carbs are not loaded with the nutrients you need. Instead, strike a balance with the number of starchy foods you consume with those high in fiber. Consume starchy carbs, such as whole grains, oats, and cereals, within the three hours after you exercise.

Fueling Before Exercise

The most important first step in calculating your nutritional timing is to determine your energy phase. This phase occurs when your body requires the most nutrients, which is often during your workout. As your energy levels deplete, the requirements for nutrition increases. So, find out the time it takes for your food to properly digest.

The secret to having enough fuel for your workout is the amount of time you let your body rest after eating. This is where nutrient timing comes into play. It is important to pack your meal with carbs, but eating too closely to the time you work out will prevent you from getting the most out of your workout. For best results, space out your eating according to the size of the meal.

If you exercise at night, plan to eat a large meal at least four hours before you hit the gym. Your body needs the time to digest the meal and appropriately absorb the nutrients received from the food consumed. Eating exactly four hours before a workout is often difficult, however, when you have a busy schedule. Cut your meal by half if you plan to work out two to three hours after you consume a meal. If you have even less time, cut that meal in half again, giving yourself a snack. The smaller amount of food allows you to work out an hour after consumption.

Timing your nutrition becomes more difficult when you work out in the mornings. After all, it is not only not recommended but bad for your body if you wake up at 2:00 AM to eat a meal and go back to sleep. Lying down soon after eating does not give your body the time it needs to digest nutrients. Instead, consider eating a larger meal at least four hours before bed. If you wake up and head straight to the gym, you should have enough energy to get you through a good workout. However, it is unwise to go without food if you are planning to work out for longer than an hour. Instead, eat a small snack before you head to the gym. Wake up a little earlier to see better benefits from taking the time to eat.

Again, fueling up before heading to the gym is highly personal. Some find eating little to nothing before a workout keeps their energy levels high while not compromising their efficiency. Others find it impossible to not eat before a meal, and doing so would cause stomach aches and other unpleasant symptoms. Map the way your body responds to fueling up by keeping a journal of your activities. If you are consistent in tracking your experience, you will find that working out is easier and more efficient than before.

Fueling Down and After Exercise

When fueling down, your goal is to prepare your body for the next exercise. So, consider what your body would need to perform well next time. Of course, your body requires protein for muscle repair and to combat soreness. Your body is also in dire need of the nutrients it lost during a difficult workout.

Common belief used to dictate that the best time to refuel is immediately after working out. The body is primed to receive nutrients because it is more receptive to insulin, making it easier for the body to break the food down better. However, studies have shown that there is a larger window than once believed. Instead of chugging a protein shake immediately after you finish working out, you have around an hour when your body is primed for optimal nutrient breakdown.

Pack your next meal with as many nutrients as you can to promote muscle and tissue repair and growth. According to health consultants Tiffani Bachus and Erin Macdonald, "For a post-workout meal, aim for 15-25 grams of protein (for tissue repair) and 1-2 grams/kg (of body weight) of carbohydrates per hour of glycogen-depleting exercise. Add 5-10 grams of fat for satiation purposes." (2017) As long as you are getting enough nutrients from eating correctly, you do not need to worry about adding supplements.

Most nutritionists have mixed reviews of eating right before bed. If you work out in the evening, it is often difficult to wait four hours after eating to go to bed. So, should you skip the meal altogether to avoid gaining fat storages while you sleep? The answer is no. Your body still needs fuel to repair its system. Robbing your body of nutrients will not only make you hungry in the middle of the night, but it could also damage your chances to build large muscles. Remember, your body requires fuel for repairs. Any fuel deprivation could cause issues in the long run.

Fueling for Rest Day

Rest day is the perfect time for your body to cope with the changes it has experienced in the last 24 hours. If your body takes longer to heal (48 hours is usually the longest it takes for slow bodies to heal), use your down time to prepare your muscles for strain by maintaining a diet that will support you. Eating is the primary reason for healthy muscle growth, so eat correctly.

Skip the sports foods on your rest day. On the days you go to the gym, you can consume protein shakes, protein bars, and pre-workout shakes, but rest days are for focusing on nutrients you can consume with meals. Eat lots of fruits and vegetables, load up on healthy proteins like chicken and fish, and get the vitamins and minerals you need for your next workout day.

The timing for eating proteins, however, is different on rest days. Instead of eating protein before a workout and immediately after, space out your protein consumption by several hours, eating 20-30 grams throughout the day. Protein is no less important on rest days.

Rest days do not mean the end of carbs, but you should be aware of the types you ingest. Try to avoid simple sugars and focus on complex carbohydrates that will give you the most bang for your buck. Instead of focusing solely on eating whole grains, change up your diet to include beans and legumes and switch bananas out for berries.

Next, how many times you eat on rest days affects how you will build muscle. If you are eating to lose weight and gain muscle, consider either slimming down the number of meals you consume. Many theories suggest you should eat either just one meal or six meals daily. Eating only one meal a day has worked for some, but cramming all your necessary nutrients into one meal is not ideal nor consistent. Eating six small meals is more doable, but the main reason you would eat so many meals is if you are training. Otherwise, stick to two to three meals daily.

If you only want to gain muscle, eat more than two meals daily. Studies have shown that eating at least 3 meals impacts muscle building positively. Ultimately, the number of meals is up to you. Many bodybuilders eat only two meals per day and drink a protein shake in the morning. Regardless of what times you eat, your ultimate goal is to give your body the nutrients it needs when you feel hungry.

How much you eat also depends on how often you rest. If you are just starting, you may only want to work out three days a week, and therefore you can consume food in smaller amounts. You should still have a relatively regular eating schedule, but it is safer to change your caloric intake every day. However, if you aim to work five or six days every week, you need to maintain a higher level of consumption. Do not consider your day off as a day to skimp on the nutrients. Eating the same amount of food on your days off will not cause you to gain significant weight. Consider what you eat as an investment in your future muscle stamina.

Rest days should be the time that you experiment with your diet. That does not mean that you should eat out at the nearest burger joint and consume massive amounts of ice cream. Instead, develop your culinary skills and shop for foods that will aid your journey to gaining muscle. Experiment with how much of each macronutrient your body needs to maintain health. Invest in storage containers to meal prep for the rest of your week, giving yourself the most energy in the most draining parts of your day.

On your off days, do not rely on caffeine to keep you awake. The body needs to rest during this critical time, and any addition to your diet that makes your body more tense than it should be requires moderation. This applies to other foods such as chocolate, alcohol, and spicy foods, just to name a few. Remember, small quantities of foods that do not help you gain muscle are acceptable when you regulate the amount.

Finally, do not forget to continue hydrating. Water is essential during exercise, but it is just as essential when not exercising. The body requires water to perform basic functions, making it the most important part of your diet. Form a habit of drinking water on a schedule, even when you feel you do not need it.

CHAPTER 4:
THE SCIENTIFIC WAY TO LOSE FAT

Many dieting gurus will tell you that there is something special in certain organic foods you consume, or that the fat you lose

is burned through expending energy. However, many of these so-called "gurus" do not know what happens to fat once you get rid of it. The science of body composition and fat content is the key to understanding how to lose fat, and for good.

The Mathematics of Weight Loss

When asked what happens to your fat during weight loss, many people do not know the answer. Where does the fat go? Many explain that fat is lost through a combination of waste and heat. When you work out, the extra fat in your body is manifested as energy and lost in a chemical reaction that burns heat. That is where the term "burning calories" comes from.

Though that sounds highly scientific, fat is not lost through chemical reactions in the body that convert fat into heat. Fat is composed of matter, and matter does not simply dissolve into thin air when the body exerts itself. No matter is lost in the universe. All matter exists from the beginning of the universe to now. Neither is fat lost through excretion.

The nutrients you put into your body do not become part of your body until they can be broken down into key elements. Your body uses what it needs and discards the rest. The body does not have use for additional fiber, which passes through the body, just as a ball would fall through the center of a pipe. The rest of the broken down material becomes fuel for future energy, and the molecules are rearranged to best suit your body.

Proteins, carbs, fats, sugars, and other macronutrients are made of three main molecular ingredients: carbon, oxygen, and hydrogen. These are the building blocks for life. The macronutrients you do not use as energy turn into fat, which is also composed of these three molecules. The matter, therefore, is not created, but rather transferred to a different form.

Fat is composed of carbon, hydrogen, and oxygen. You may remember from high school chemistry that the majority of what we breathe out is carbon dioxide, or CO_2, and water is defined with two hydrogen and one oxygen, or H_2O. What we breathe in, on the other hand, is composed of the same molecules but rearranged in the form of fat, which is $C_{55}H_{104}O_6$. Though the amount of carbon and hydrogen atoms may fluctuate, you will always see the same number of oxygen molecules in fat. Our bodies are designed to consume fat and oxygen and release carbon dioxide and water.

Exercise helps you lose fat, but how does it work? Fat is a hefty molecule, made of approximately 55 carbons atoms, 104 hydrogen, and 6 of oxygen (hence the $C_{55}H_{104}o_6$ numeration). Strenuous activity helps the proteins in your body break down the fat into the carbon dioxide and water. When you breathe out, you are breathing away the atoms that once composed the fat in your body.

Many people become vastly confused by this because carbon dioxide and water molecules that exit the body are invisible. They only appear as solids at extremely low temperatures, which makes it difficult to picture how fat is lost. So, exercising at high levels causes your body to exert more force and produce more air, effectively ridding your body of the extra carbon, hydrogen, and oxygen molecules.

But, it hardly seems likely that most or even half of the compounds that leave your body are composed of water. If that were the case, your breath would be a lot wetter. So, what is the composition of water and carbon dioxide that leaves the body when releasing fat? If you are a science buff, you will notice that stoichiometry (the relationship between relative quantities of substances) dictates that the number of molecules that are part of a chemical reaction must be equal on either side of the equation. That means that there are as many molecules of carbon, hydrogen, and oxygen from a combination of fat and oxygen as there are of carbon dioxide and water when the reaction is complete. The resulting balanced equation is as follows.

To calculate the correct ratio of carbon dioxide and water expended when burning fat, consider the oxygens. As you will notice, there are twice as many oxygens available in carbon dioxide than there are in water. Therefore, carbon dioxide molecules are the most common leaving the body. Calculating the masses of carbon, oxygen, and hydrogen associated with each gives the following equations.

Since there are six oxygens associated with a fat molecule and there are twice as many oxygens in carbon dioxide as there are in water, four oxygens are included in the carbon equation, and two are located with hydrogens, giving the following equations.

The resulting percentage of each molecule leaving the body is given by 84% and 16% . So, the majority of fat leaving the body is invisible to the naked eye. The more you breathe out when exercising, the more fat is ultimately lost.

Many get confused when discussing calories after this breakdown. After all, calories provide the body with energy. However, as mentioned previously, the official definition of a calorie is the energy it takes to increase the temperature of 1 kg of water. The energy, therefore, is expended during metabolization of foods. The heat you experience is the result of a chemical reaction.

All energy that you get from foods comes from the sun. Think about it: plants produce chlorophyll, a substance that converts sunlight into molecules. Many animals eat plants almost exclusively, which then gives them the basic molecules mentioned previously: carbon, hydrogen, and oxygen. In essence, when you eat, you are eating sunlight.

Many so-called "gurus" will tell you that there is a secret formula to losing weight that can only be achieved through taking supplements or pills that only they can provide. Before you get caught up in the hype, consider how these supplements will magically cause your weight to lift off of your body. If they do not know how fat is expended, it is highly unlikely that they will know how to create a supplement that will take care of the weight loss for you.

The science for losing weight is very simple: all you have to do is breathe more and eat less. So, if you sit on a couch all day and simply breathe as quickly as you can you will lose weight just as easily as those who work out daily, right? Sitting still does not cause hormones in the body to break down the fat cells in your body. Insulin and testosterone, among some others, are released during exercise allowing for the breakdown of the cells. Fat cells do not break down on their own, and only the energy they store is for the body to naturally produce hormones.

When you eat less, your body does not have the opportunity to send as many molecules to storage, preventing the buildup of fat cells. The nutrients you do consume will be used for your benefit throughout the day, and eating less than you expend forces the body to turn to its own energy sources. Breaking down fat is not easy, and the body uses other sources of energy first, but you will experience fat loss when you combine your expenditure of breath with less dependence on food.

When to Lose Weight

When you feel as though you are suffering from physical inabilities or if you simply do not like the way you look in the mirror because of excess weight, it is time to consider losing weight. The way to do this has been preached for years: eat less and exercise more. However, there is more to weight loss than wanting to lose weight. It also comes down to timing. When is the best time to focus on weight loss?

There are two distinct times to focus on weight loss: before and after muscle gain. Attempting to lose weight while you gain muscle often leads to frustration and the inability to maintain a healthy schedule. Losing fat and gaining muscle at the same time may seem like the perfect way to multitask, but you will not see results as quickly, which will prevent you from making the right exercise and eating choices. To see the most results and keep yourself from frustration, stick with losing weight either before or after you gain muscle.

Before Muscle Gain

If it is clear that you want to lose weight based on health or personal reasons, consider losing weight before you gain muscle. Muscle will develop under fat, and if you lose fat at the same rate that you gain muscle, the scale will not budge. It is also difficult to see the results of your hard work. This option is a great way to start your journey to a shredded body.

The best way to remove fat before starting an intense muscle-building routine is to create a deficit in your caloric intake. Use the chart from Chapter 1 to determine how many calories you should eat every day and subtract 500. Do not follow the hype that you need to lose weight at a greater caloric loss than that. Remember, your body still needs nutrients to heal from exercise and to prevent low energy.

When you become comfortable with eating 500 calories less than you currently do, you can progressively lower that number, stopping at 1000 calories below your average calorie consumption. Find your comfort zone when eating fewer calories, and eat when you get hungry. Make sure to wait for that feeling of hunger before you consider eating again. Staying consistent with this pattern will help you lose weight in a healthy and sustainable way. Eating disorders often form when you believe you cannot reach your goal and become frustrated; this simple plan isn't about deprivation and impossible goals. So, remember to treat yourself every so often to reward yourself and not become frustrated while dieting.

Next, calculate the number of calories you burn during exercise and halve it. The new number is the number of calories you can add to your diet. Exercise does not give you the excuse to eat more. In fact, that is where many dieters hit a rough patch, believing that they deserve to overcompensate for the calories lost. Your body will still retain the amount of nutrients it needs when working out, but you will see greater strides in fat loss when you follow this plan.

Before each meal, consume two glasses of water. Remember that sugary drinks have empty calories, so avoid them before meals. Thirst can mask itself as hunger, which often causes you to eat instead of drink. When you are thirsty, you are more likely to feel a sudden pang in your stomach, but true feelings of hunger manifest themselves as slow aches that build throughout the day. Do not be fooled into thinking that you are hungry when you are actually thirsty.

Consuming water fills up the stomach. Drinking water even when you are hungry has serious benefits, and you will notice that you are less anxious to eat after drinking two glasses of water. Cravings for sugary and salty foods are also often curbed by drinking water. The dreaded "munchy" phase (when you are not really hungry but want to eat something) loses its power when you drink water. So, the next time you reach for a donut, consider downing a bottle of water instead.

When dishing up food, put it on a smaller plate. The mind plays tricks on the body when it is used to behaving in the same way. When you see a small helping of food on a large plate, you feel as though you are not getting the nutrients you need. Many severely underestimate the number of calories they consume every day, and making your food look smaller than it is plays a part in the deception. Instead, use a small plate and pile on the same amount of food. Suddenly, the meal looks like it has significantly increased in size, and you can trick your body into believing that you are getting more food than you are.

Eat your food slower. You are more likely to feel full when you take your time to chow down on food. Think of the last time you were hungry and scarfed down mountains of food. It is likely that you did not realize that you were full until you had let your food settle. Then, you realized you ate too much and you feel full and bloated. Eating slowly not only helps you feel full sooner, but you can enjoy the taste longer. Chew at least ten times before swallowing to help in digestion and mindfully let yourself acknowledge the calories you are consuming.

Plan your meals and develop an eating schedule. Many people use storage containers to divide their food throughout the day, and that might just be the key to getting the most out of your diet. If you are more comfortable following a three-meal eating schedule, do it. However, if you get hungrier between meals, it might be better to increase your number of meals while decreasing the size. Give yourself a snack in between meals to give yourself more energy and prevent hunger. You are more likely to overeat when you are hungry, so satisfy your hunger without going overboard. Eat low-calorie snacks when you start to feel cravings coming on. Carrots and celery are excellent choices because they are low in calories and give a satisfying crunch.

Another way to combat cravings is to imagine eating the food you want. Though it may seem like torture at first, it actually trains the brain to receive pleasure from hormone release instead of eating unhealthy foods. When a craving occurs, close your eyes and imagine yourself eating it for 30 seconds. You will fool your brain into thinking your craving has been satisfied.

Keep yourself away from snack foods by not letting them into the house. If you see snacks, you are more likely to instinctively reach for them. It becomes much more difficult when others bring those snacks home. Make a rule to prohibit as many snacks as you can. Instead, save sugary snacks for outside the house. Go out for an ice cream cone or enjoy time in a bakery with friends. Train your brain to stop craving foods when you are at home.

Cardio is helpful when losing weight, but it is not a requirement. Many choose to add cardio to their exercise routines because it increases your heart rate and breathing rate. Your weight changes over time when losing fat, so you may experience lengthening of muscles and an increase in lean muscle.

Adding cardio to your routine helps you in other ways as well. Running has been proven to combat depression and anxiety by increasing "happy hormones" such as dopamine and serotonin. So, though it is not necessary to lose fat, it does give you the motivation to continue exercising before you start building muscle. It will also get you in the habit of exercising several days each week. Though rest days are important, it is possible to exercise more often when performing cardio.

If you are just starting cardio, gradually work up to more time on the treadmill or on the road. Your joints will not receive the same impact on the treadmill that they will on the road, so if you suffer from aching bones after running, consider visiting the gym. Start alternating running and walking in one minute intervals and gradually increase the number of minutes of running until you have reached half an hour to 45 minutes. Many people can manage adding another minute of running to their routines every time they hit the gym.

After Muscle Gain

Losing fat is more difficult after you begin a muscle-building routine. Your body needs extra nutrients to gain and maintain muscle, which means it is more difficult for the fat to break down when you are eating more. Also, when you have gained a significant portion of muscle, it is more likely that you will lose muscle and fat weight at the same rate. Therefore, losing weight after gaining muscle is only recommended for people who have already mastered their diets.

For best results, aim to lose 0.7% of your body fat every week (Shapiro, n.d.-a). Approximately 3500 calories equal one pound of fat. So, calculate the calorie deficit to make this happen. Remember, a majority of the calories you burn are expended during regular bodily operations like breathing, so you do not have to kill yourself getting rid of those extra calories.

Double the amount of protein you consume when losing fat and gaining muscle. Protein is responsible for repairing and building muscle, so your body must focus primarily on using the protein instead of storing it for later. Since it is wise to eat approximately 0.36 grams for every pound you weigh, double that figure to 0.72. That means that, if you weigh 150 pounds, you should consume 108 grams of protein. Tie that number into the number of calories you eat every day, and you might realize that much of your diet is already accounted for.

The next step is to reduce carbs. Carbs give your body temporary energy in your muscles, so do not get rid of them altogether, however. Instead, find a healthy alternative to starches such as pasta and potatoes by choosing fats or proteins that will fit the bill. Remember, do not be afraid of eating carbs, proteins, or fats, as each provides your body with energy and can be used effectively when broken down during exercise.

When completing your food journal for your workout days, eat all the calories your diet allows. If you do not eat all the macronutrients you need during the day, your fat may decrease, but it is often also at the expense of your muscle weight. Starving yourself will not allow your muscles to build themselves stronger. Going overboard on your caloric intake on off days is detrimental to fat loss as well. All the nutrients you do not use will be converted to fat.

Your non-workout days may seem like the perfect days to stay on the couch and munch on your favorite snack, but you may still work out during off days. In fact, it is encouraged. Instead of focusing on building muscle, perform high-intensity interval training (HIIT), which forces your body to expend energy to achieve simple tasks for short intervals. Though it may not seem like much, HIIT gives your body the extra boost it needs when working out without putting too much strain on your muscles.

Preserving Healthy Muscle During Weight Loss

Those who struggle with obesity do not have an absence of muscle. Studies have shown that obesity is instead a problem with muscle composition. The muscles in an obese person do not perform to their full potential, resulting in weakness. It should be no surprise, then, that the poor muscle makes small tasks, like walking up stairs, difficult.

Those past the age of 50 are more commonly impacted by these results than younger people. Muscles start to significantly decrease in size from the age of 50 onward if not properly maintained. Simple tasks such as lifting an object to a high shelf or walking on uneven ground may result in falls because of poor muscle quality. The harder it becomes to grip well, the more likely it is that your muscles are losing integrity. It is for this reason that many institutions now focus on the quality of muscles rather than gaining muscle when aging.

Weight loss is important to those with obesity for many reasons, including the loss of fat. However, creating a caloric intake deficit, you also run the risk of losing fat-free mass, which is essentially muscle. However, this should not alarm you. The poor quality of muscles for people with obesity means that the muscles contain too many layers, preventing proteins from working efficiently. When you lose muscle mass due to healthy dieting, you are losing inefficient parts of the muscle.

Many people who take the "easy" approach to weight loss (losing it through bariatric surgery) often find that their results do not tend to stick after one to two years after receiving the surgery. This, in a large part, has to do with the effectiveness of muscles to maintain weight. Since the quantity instead of the quality of muscles were changed, the weight does not stay off forever.

So, the recommended way to get rid of fat is to lose body mass while preventing the loss of significant non-fat mass. The best way to achieve this is through brisk, moderate to high-intensity workout sessions for an average of 300 minutes every week. Studies have shown that it is possible to lose weight by only creating a deficit in the number of calories you consume daily, but your body will be more prone to adapt to consistent weight loss when building muscle.

A combination of muscle building, endurance training, and a healthy diet is the best way to lose weight. When you build muscle, you are forcing your muscles to change. They will knit together tighter and eventually grow larger. Endurance training forces the muscles to maintain a high level of compression for long periods of time, further refining them.

Both those who whittle their bodies down to smaller sizes through exercise and those who receive bariatric surgery also show an increased amount of weight loss associated with a higher intake of protein. Though only a small increase in protein is required to get the most out of your diet, that little bit is significantly important. Protein is required to prevent fat-free mass loss. Instead of eating away at your body reducing the number of calories you consume, when paired with exercise, this additional amount of protein you consume promotes the loss of fat while maintaining muscle.

CHAPTER 5:
VITAMINS, MINERALS, AND SUPPLEMENTS YOU NEED

Eating the right kinds of foods, the right amount of food, and eating it at the right time provides you with everything you need, right? Well, if you have spent a lot of time working out, you will realize that you do not always get what you need from the foods you consume. Though it is not always necessary to take additional vitamins, minerals, and supplements, their addition to your diet could help you perform and feel better when you head to the gym.

Chapter 1 briefly covered some vitamins, minerals, and supplements that are important to building muscle, but this chapter takes a closer view of them and offers a few more for consideration. Ultimately your health is dependent on how well you feel consuming the macronutrients you do, so slight adjustments or foregoing some of these options altogether may be your best option. Make sure to consult your doctor to find which supplements you can or cannot take based on your daily diet.

The Only 3 Top Muscle-Building Supplements

When you are headed to the gym, it is nice to know that you will have all the right tools in your arsenal. But, how do you know exactly which supplements to take that will help you build more muscle? There are so many conflicting reviews regarding which are the best supplements to take when building muscle, but the best comes from natural sources simply accentuated with additional supplementation.

Protein

The top of any muscle-building list is protein. As we've discussed, it is responsible for creating and repairing muscle, and is one of the most important nutritional supplements to take when gaining muscle. It should be no secret, then, that it is often required to ingest more protein that is available in an everyday diet. Luckily, many stores provide affordable options to give you the extra protein you need. A common way to consume protein is through powder because it gives you the necessary protein for muscle growth without unnecessary additives. These are found in many forms including whey protein, rice protein, and pea protein.

Whey protein is commonly found in milk, but its powder alternative allows those with lactose intolerance to consume it without repercussions. Studies have shown that whey protein aids in weight fat loss as well. Paired with a 500 calorie deficit diet, subjects who consumed whey protein showed a significant loss of fat compared to those who did not (Frestedt et al., 2008). The study also showed that the addition of muscle-gaining exercise added to the final weight loss results. Whey protein is also responsible for lowering the risk of cancer, lowering cholesterol, and treating asthma.

Despite the belief that rice is simply a carb, it does contain significant amounts of protein, which makes it an excellent source for people who try to avoid meat products. The proteins that come from rice proteins have approximately the same effects as whey protein. A study conducted with MMA fighters as the subjects comparing whey and rice proteins reported the same amount of muscle gain and weight loss for both. Rice protein, however, is not considered a full protein because it does not contain all amino acids in protein. Lysine is the only amino acid absent. However, you can find this amino acid in other animal products.

Pea protein, like rice protein, comes from plants. Pea plants are crushed into a powder, leaving mostly protein behind. While pea protein is also not a complete protein, it contains all the amino acids necessary, but it does not have enough methionine+cysteine to be considered a full protein. It also contains a high dose of iron, a supplement necessary to help your body function well in stressful situations. Pea protein is an excellent alternative to whey and rice protein because it offers all the same benefits without bloating. It is also a highly beneficial weight-loss supplement because it causes the body to feel full.

Like mentioned previously, protein is mostly abundant in everyday meals, so it is often unnecessary to add too much protein to your diet. Check the food you eat every day to get a better feeling of how much protein to consume. Most people get at least 30% of the necessary protein from consuming food, if not more (Shapiro, n.d.-a). If you eat a lot of meat, you may find that there is very little to add to your diet.

There is no specific time of day to consume protein supplements. But, as I've said, do not consume protein within the four hours before you go to bed. Other than that, the choice is completely yours. Many take protein within the first hour after a workout. Try consuming protein at this time and judge its effects. There is no scientific evidence that states that is the proper time to take the supplement, but it is highly variable with how your body reacts to the supplement.

Creatine

Creatine, in and of itself, does not create muscles. In fact, it has little to do with the building of muscles except for its effects on energy in the body. Creatine gives your body extra energy to work harder and longer. So, though creatine does not directly influence the way your muscles grow, it does allow you to work harder, which helps you build muscle.

Creatine increases the capacity for your muscles to create ATP, which is energy created in the body. Your body can only create so much ATP at one time, and it is often insufficient for hard workouts. Creatine is naturally found in the body, but it is often in limited supply. This is why you feel tired after working at a high rate. Therefore, taking a creatine supplement will help the body overcome its threshold by activating more ATP in the body. Creatine is often linked to increased muscle mass over long periods of time. Creatine aids in adding water to the muscles and improving protein metabolism.

Creatine is recommended in three to five grams of daily consumption and is found at many drug stores that sell supplements. Consult your doctor before starting a creatine routine to avoid side effects. Also, women tend to show less favorable effects than men when taking the supplement; it offers little additional help to building muscle. The supplement is most found in a powder form that is available at any drug store. Though not everyone benefits from creatine, it is inexpensive and generally safe to use, so it is worth trying.

Aim for ingesting creatine at the same time as protein supplements. Though it is not necessary to do so, it does save you time and aids in developing a habit of consuming it every day. If you are just starting, specialists suggest that you take four times the regular amount to saturate your body with creatine. So, if the supplement suggests you take 5 g of creatine every day, take 5 g four times a day for one week to introduce it into your system. It is recommended that the supplement be taken with food, so add it to your meals.

Citrulline Malate

Finally, citrulline malate is another common supplement that aids in your performance. That said, it does not necessarily help your muscles grow faster, only aiding your body in completing more reps at the gym. This endurance booster is not necessary, but it can be helpful to some.

Since citrulline malate does not naturally occur in the body, nor are there many significant amounts of it in food, there is a limited number of studies completed on the supplement. However, it has been noted that those who use it often experience a boost in endurance and power output. This supplement also does not have enough studies to suggest that it provides serious drawbacks. For those who take the supplement, they do not report any side effects.

It is not necessary to take citrulline malate every day. In fact, it is recommended to keep it out of your diet if you are not working out. So, consuming the supplement on off days and consumption far before a workout are not recommended. Instead, wait until an hour before your workout to take it. Take approximately three grams before your workouts.

Top 4 Muscle-Building Nutrients That Aren't Protein

Protein is massively important to building muscle. From repairing to rebuilding muscle, nothing works quite as well as protein. However, that does not mean that there are not other supplements that are equally important. Building muscle has been shortened into a science, which means that we now know which vitamins, minerals, and supplements are most important to the body to get the body you are trying to achieve.

Calcium

Calcium is the most common mineral in our bodies. It is part of your bones, teeth, blood, muscle, and the fluid between every one of your billions of cells (Muscle and Strength, n.d.). So, those who suffer from calcium deficiencies cannot perform well. Diseases, such as osteoporosis, are just the tip of the iceberg concerning problems related to calcium deficiencies. Without calcium, your body cannot effectively send impulses to the brain, so your responses are slower. Your body can also not activate satellite cells in your muscles when you have a calcium deficiency, which makes gaining muscle difficult.

Though there is a slight discrepancy related the amount of calcium you should consume every day depending on sex and age, it is recommended to consume at least one gram of calcium every day. Since calcium is highly abundant in nature, it is not difficult to get your calcium from the food you consume. Dairy is the main source of calcium for many in the world, which includes milk, cheese, and yogurt. However, if you are a vegan, kale and broccoli are also excellent sources from the vegetable family. Fish and most grains also contain some amounts of calcium, though they do not constitute a significant source. Still, you can consume what you need from these sources by ingesting them in large amounts. Finally, many cereals and fruit juices include some calcium due enrichment of this mineral.

Most of the calcium supplements you can buy are found in daily multivitamins. Other over the counter sources often require you to eat and drink something when taking them for the best results. Calcium carbonate is the most common form of supplement, but it often requires that you take food with it. Tums is a common source for calcium carbonate. Calcium citrate is another form of calcium supplement that is usually more expensive than its calcium carbonate counterpart. It is easier for most people to absorb this form of calcium, and it does not require you to eat food when taking it.

Though calcium is highly necessary to daily diets, remember that it is possible to add too much to your diet. This often gives you the opposite effect of what calcium usually does for your body. Too much calcium may result in weakened bones and kidney stones. Initial signs, however, are often manifested as bloating, gas, and constipation. If you are experiencing any of these symptoms, stop taking the supplement and consult a doctor.

Though anyone can have a calcium deficiency, there are some who are more likely to experience it than others. Postmenopausal women often experience calcium insufficiency because it is difficult for their bodies to break down the source. Women who experience a stop in menstruation are also prone to calcium loss. When their menstruation stops, it is often a sign that they are not getting the right amount of calcium. Those who suffer from lactose intolerance often do not get enough calcium because they cannot ingest dairy. Similarly, vegans also suffer from a loss of calcium due to the inability to access foods with high levels of calcium.

Vitamin D

Vitamin D is often associated with the sun, but many foods also contain it. Vitamin D is also responsible for keeping bones strong, and it is often paired with calcium. Without vitamin D, bones become brittle, which is associated with rickets in children and osteoporosis in adults. Vitamin D is also responsible for maintaining a healthy immune system. You may notice that, if during the winter months, it is easier to become sick. While not all of this is responsible for a lack of vitamin D, the vitamin does allow the body to better combat sickness. It is also considered one of the building blocks of human growth and development.

It's generally recommended to consume 400 mg of vitamin D every day, regardless of age or sex. It is more difficult, however, to naturally consume more vitamin D. Many of the products at the market that boast of containing large amounts of vitamin D actually use a supplement. Fatty fish, however, are a natural source of vitamin D, which include mackerel, tuna, and salmon. Beef, eggs, and cheese also contain trace amounts, though you would need to consume them in large amounts to receive the benefits. Many cereals and orange juices also contain added vitamin D.

Sunlight, of course, is the ultimate source of vitamin D, but spending many hours in the sun can have its own problems. UV light can cause skin cancer and other damage to the skin. Tanning beds, which are also commonly used to get enough vitamin D, also pose some of the same risks. Those who wear clothing covering their skin or sunscreen will not receive the same benefits of gaining vitamin D that others will, so aim for spending some time in the sun, but not overdoing it.

Many do not receive the benefits of vitamin D based on their location or skin color. Darker-skinned people do not receive as much of the vitamin as those of lighter skins because their bodies do not absorb the nutrient at a high rate. Those with lighter skin often receive more vitamin D when out in the sun because ancestry has dictated that they will receive less sunlight than those of darker skins. It is highly unlikely that you will have too much vitamin D in your diet, so consider including it via limited sun exposure.

It is also common for older adults to not receive the right amount of vitamin D every day. This is due to the inefficiencies of getting older. As we age, our bodies can't convert vitamin D from sunlight, putting us at risk of not having enough to maintain healthy levels.

HMB

Hydroxymethylbutyrate (HMB) is responsible for breaking down the leucine, an amino acid. It aids in preventing muscle breakdown, and thus is a common supplement for muscle builders. Studies have shown that HMB aids in keeping muscles active during down time. HMB has become a popular ingredient in many medicines today, making it a hot item.

HMB is commonly used for people who build muscle because, especially at older ages, the body becomes more likely to lose muscle. This muscle-maintenance supplement is ideal for people over 50 years old. It is included in many protein shakes, so be sure to read the labels when shopping.

Take HMB with food, and do so before working out. The recommended dosage is one to three grams every day. If you find that three grams is the best dosage for you, space it out across three meals and throughout the day. Also, take the supplement 30-45 minutes before working out.

Zinc

You may have noticed zinc in drug stores along with other vitamins and minerals. This is because it is essential to growth, muscle repair, and aids the immune system. Zinc is responsible for growth for all age groups, especially in children. Zinc aids in building proteins for the body, making it irreplaceable when building muscle.

Far lower than the amounts for many other vitamins and minerals, the body requires a daily consumption of 8 - 13 mg. The best source of zinc in food comes from oysters. However, if you do not have constant access to oysters, beef, poultry, and seafood are excellent sources as well. Vegans can consume beans, whole grains, and nuts, which provide a lower source of zinc. Other foods, such as breakfast cereals, are enhanced with zinc.

Zinc is also available as oral supplements in drug stores, and it is commonly available in multivitamins. It is not necessary to purchase the zinc supplement alone; many supplement formulas contain mixtures of calcium and magnesium along with zinc. Other sources, such as denture cream and nasal sprays, also contain trace amounts of the mineral, but be aware of the risks. You may temporarily experience a loss of smell or taste after using these products. That does not mean that are unsafe, only that zinc has unique interactions with the senses.

A lack of zinc in the body has negative effects that you should address immediately. Those with little zinc in their systems are often sick because the mineral aids the immune system. Some studies have reported that using a liquid form of zinc, such as cough syrup, may recover from simple colds as well. Many who are malnourished also suffer from a lack of zinc consumption, resulting in diarrhea. This condition can become life threatening if not treated properly.

Zinc's effects when in too high dosages can have the same effects. When the body is overloaded with zinc, the immune system often struggles. You might also experience nausea, diarrhea, loss of appetite, stomach aches, and headaches. The recommended dosage of zinc is minimal, so consult a doctor before using this supplement.

Performance Enhancers and Herbs

Performance enhancers and herbs have become increasingly popular over the years, and their numbers of sales continue to climb. These herbs are natural, plant-based supplements that claim to boost athletic performance. However, there is very little evidence to back up the fact that these herbs benefit athletes, especially since there are a wide variety of factors. Many athletes self-medicate, which means it is nearly impossible to gain solid evidence that a herb does what it claims to do.

Still, members of the athletic community find interest in a variety of herbs, echinacea and ginseng among the most prevalent now. Despite the wide variety of factors that might influence the effectiveness of these herbs, such as production, storage, and consumption, athletes often swear by their performative powers.

Why Athletes Use Herbs

Athletes who perform rigorous routines with little to no support from supplements often suffer from sickness more often than those with a sedentary lifestyle. Those who claim to work out a moderate amount (30 minutes a few days a week) often see the benefits of their training by showing less susceptibility to these effects. It is only the truly intensely trained athletes that suffer from the overload of work. The extra stressors on the body are difficult to withstand, especially during difficult training. To combat some of these effects, athletes turn to herbs and performance enhancers.

Popular Herbs

Since popular herbs are not considered part of an "other" category, there is little scientific backing to taking these herbs. For the most part, these herbs benefit one part of the body, like the central nervous system for ginseng and immune system capabilities for echinacea.

The purported results make taking these alternative herbs more popular.

Echinacea is reported to help the upper respiratory system, which is usually under attack when subjecting the body to rigorous routines. White blood cells are responsible for the majority of immune health, to which echinacea is reportedly associated. However, two studies done on the herb found that there was little to no change in the white blood cell count after four weeks of athletic participant consumption. However, they were able to determine that the subjects did suffer from less upper-respiratory system illnesses than those not taking the herb. In conclusion, they associated the herb with aiding in changing white blood cells, making them more capable of fighting infections. The increase in oxygen consumption and retention associated with echinacea supports this theory.

There are nine total species of echinacea, and each has a different effect on the human body. Studies performed by David Senchina determined that each athlete who added the supplement to his or her diet showed remarkable changes in the oxygen levels and versatility of white blood cells. Participants were taken from a wide variety of athletes, including soccer players and runners, and even the type of sport often yielded varied results. However, each showed an improvement in immune capability compared with the control group.

Echinacea's effectiveness is highly dependent on its production and the subject's athletic background. Studies have shown that even a small change in the production often leads to mixed results. Different manufacturers or even bundles may exhibit wild changes in results. The amount of exercise also has a large influence on the effectiveness of the herb, often showing little results in those who do not exercise often and increasing in strength for those that perform more often.

Ginseng is primarily used for performance enhancement, but the results of its efficiency are often varied. Studies conducted on the effectiveness of the herb were often inconclusive. Batches of ginseng, like echinacea, often vary, making it difficult to pin down the effectiveness of the herb. However, the side effects of taking ginseng often result in insomnia and negative interactions with other prescription drugs.

When compared to echinacea, ginseng does not hold the same level of effectiveness. The results of affecting the immune system were also inconclusive, displaying spikes in effectiveness. Ginseng is more popular in the United States than echinacea, but it does not have the same promising results. Other factors that influence its effectiveness are an athlete's age, sex, and exercise routine. Since there are also a number of ginseng variations, it is difficult to determine which is most effective.

Do You Need Supplements?

Some supplements are highly helpful to get you the results you want, but they are hardly necessary. In fact, if you only consume water and a good diet, you will still see results. However, some like the effects of supplements to the diet, and it may result in better health. The effects of taking supplements are noted in this chapter, so it is up to you to do your own research on the subject and find which are best for you.

The most effective way to gain muscle is to perform exercises correctly and follow a good diet. Though you may see people at the gym who perform hundreds of repetitions while staring in the mirror, only those who do the work properly will see the results. The supplements you take will help to stimulate muscle growth, but you will not reap the benefits if you do not put in the work.

Choosing a Sensible Approach to Enhance Exercise and Athletic Performance

The best way to determine which supplements you need are to contact your doctor and experiment. Remember, taking supplements is highly personal, and some might work better than others. Many choose to take more supplements as they age, and women are more likely than men to take these supplements. Athletes are also more likely to take supplements than those with sedentary lifestyles. It all depends on what helps you build muscle and feel well.

Supplements are most effective when paired with a healthy diet, so do not use them as a replacement for food. For example, lifting weights for long periods of time and increasing the levels at which you work will often require you to drink more water and add more electrolytes to your body. If you are not getting enough of a vitamin or mineral in your diet, change your diet first.

CHAPTER 6:
THE ULTIMATE PLAN TO BUILD MUSCLE

Once you start your journey to gaining muscle, you must maintain a healthy diet and workout routine that will sustain you as your body continues to experience consistent strain. Do not fall into the trap that you must destroy your body physically by eating too little or working out too much to see your body change rapidly. Though you may see results quicker, it is impossible to maintain this lifestyle, and your body will revert to its previous state. The best way to gain muscle is through consistent hard work.

If you are just starting your muscle building journey, it can be overwhelming. But, this chapter gives you everything you need to start and maintain a healthy muscle-building routine. The ultimate goal of this plan is to gain muscle and lose fat, giving you a healthy transformation while giving you the body you always wanted.

How to Pack Your Kitchen

Part of building your best body is building your best nutritional background. That means the first part of your journey starts in the kitchen. Eating should not be a burden, neither should it be atrociously boring. To achieve the proper diet, all you need to do is follow some simple rules.

The first step to building your best body is stocking your kitchen with healthy supplies to help you maintain energy. As discussed previously, it is important to have protein, carbs, and fats, but how much of each do you need, and what are the best options for consumption?

Let's take a look at that, now.

Starches

Whichever way you spin it, you cannot get the results you want without eating carbs. They contain the essential molecules that make up the components of our bodies: carbon, oxygen, and hydrogen. These break down into glucose, which is essentially the fuel of the body. So, the best way to fuel your body when working out is to add the right kinds of carbs that help your body the most.

Foods like oats, beans, and whole grains are optimal for giving you the right amount of blood sugar. Unlike sugars added to the diet, these starches allow your body to slowly break the food down, giving you a gentle rise in blood sugar without dumping it on you all at once. One third of your caloric intake should include starchy products, according to the Foods Standard Agency (Men's Health, 2014). Aim for foods such as whole grain bread to get the most glucose per meal.

Ingesting carbs is the only way for the body to get fiber, which is why eating more carbs than any other type of food is absolutely essential. Without it, the body cannot break down some nutrients, causing constipation. Many vegetables provide you a large dose of fiber to your diet.

When you need enough energy to build muscle, your first stop should be your starch supply. Naturally, sugary starches allow your body to maintain energy while working out. Bananas are an excellent source for sugary starches. Rebuilding muscle also requires a healthy dose of carbs, as carbs, proteins, and fats are needed to effectively aid in repair. Supplies like chocolate milk fill all of those requirements and give you a treat after working out.

Starches like blueberries are also effective in maintaining brain health. You may have noticed that a low-carb diet often leaves you feeling sluggish or poorly motivated. However, by increasing your intake of carbs by eating berries, you could feel an increase in brain power. Glucose is needed for both the body and brain, and starches give your body these benefits in small doses. Have the following starches in your pantry.

- Quinoa
- Brown rice
- Red and yellow potatoes
- Strawberries
- Bananas
- Whole grains
- Sweet potatoes

Protein

Of course, no list would be complete without mentioning the protein needed to maintain a healthy diet. They are largely responsible for gains in muscle mass and repair, but what kinds of protein should you ingest? Some are better than others, of course, because they contain leaner meat and do not include unnecessary fats. Try to look for pure proteins when stocking the kitchen.

Protein shakes such as whey protein are at the top of the list of the purest form of protein. However, not every protein powder contains the same number of nutrients. Before you select any whey protein on the shelf, inspect the ingredients to determine if it contains extra sugars and empty calories. The best brands offer a breakdown of all the ingredients and macronutrients inside.

Fish is an excellent source of protein, and it is a source of lean meat. Seafood and river fish are excellent sources of protein and provide the body with necessary macronutrients not often found in other meats such as potassium, omega-3 fatty acids, and antioxidants. Fish such as trout, salmon, and tuna each offer three to six grams of protein per serving without also consuming massive amounts of fat.

Beef is one of the most common forms of protein on the market, and it is easy to see why. Not only is it delicious, but it packs a punch in the protein department. Some cuts of beef are better for protein than others, however. If you look at the nutritional levels of different cuts of beef, you will notice a shocking variation in nutritional value. Some cuts of beef provide nearly 100% pure protein, while others, such as rib eye steaks, offer a nearly 1:1 ratio of fat to protein.

Eggs are an excellent source of protein and contain many additional nutrients that are beneficial to a healthy diet such as zinc, vitamin D, and iron. Many people, however, do not get the full benefits of eggs because they choose to forgo eating the yolk. Eggs contain both good and bad cholesterol, so eating the yolk is not harmful. You will also get more nutrients from eating the whole egg.

If you are looking for a protein that will break down over time instead of giving you a quick punch, choose cottage cheese. Many muscle builders choose this snack for nighttime to give their bodies some nutrition slowly. Also, consider adding these proteins to your diet.

- Chicken and turkey
- Lentils and other legumes/beans

- Soy proteins
- Plant-based proteins

Fruits and Vegetables

Fruits and vegetables are part of a balanced diet because they offer the body low-fat nutrients, natural sugars, and carbs. They also offer the body needed vitamins and minerals not found in other carb, protein, and fat sources. Multivitamins may be good supplements, but they do not give all the nutrients needed for a healthy diet.

Mangoes, for instance, are high in potassium, phosphorus, and calcium, giving the body excellent sources of the food without additives. However, mangoes have a slightly higher caloric count than many other fruits. Pomegranates, on the other hand, have gained popularity for their nutritional value without the same high number of calories. They are also rich in most of the B vitamins, vitamin K, fiber, and potassium, making them a highly beneficial fruit to add to your diet.

Blueberries and raspberries are also wildly popular for fitness nuts. One of the reasons is because of their taste, and other for their nutritional values. They contain a healthy amount of vitamin C, vitamin K, and folate to boot. Many athletes add these to a few hours before a workout to receive enough energy and boost nutrition.

Many grit their teeth when discussing kale and Brussels sprouts. They are often considered bitter and are low on the totem pole for most-desired vegetables of the year. However, Brussels sprouts and kale are some of the most popular vegetables in the fitness scene because they are healthy and give the body an edge when working out. Kale contains omega-3 fatty acids, copper, fiber, and potassium, among a slew of other benefits. Brussels sprouts contain folate, manganese, and omega-3 fatty acids, helping the body detox. Since there are many types of kale, try several varieties to find out which one you enjoy the most.

If nothing else, your kitchen should be stocked with broccoli. It contains enough vitamins K and C in a cup to last you all day. Muscle builders love this vegetable because it is highly nutritious, packing a lot in such a small package.

Other recommended fruits and vegetables are listed below.

- Beans (also acts as a source of protein)
- Avocado
- Legumes like peas and lentils (again, also a great source of protein)
- Artichoke
- Spinach
- Bell peppers
- Oranges
- Guava

Fats

Fats have gotten a bad rap for being the cause of diseases like heart disease and cancer, but not all fats are bad. In fact, if you do not eat enough fats, you will not have the ability to gain muscle as effectively. Adding a healthy amount of fats to your diet will increase testosterone levels, making gaining muscle easier.

Some of the best fats are found in animal products. Beef and dairy are common sources of whole fats that will allow you to gain muscle better. Other fats that are considered healthy are macadamia nuts, coconut oil, avocado, and extra-virgin olive oil.

The kinds of fats to avoid are trans fats. These include bakery items like donuts, vegetable shortening, non-dairy creamers, and fried fast food. These are ultimately responsible for diseases when consumed in large quantities. The best fats are listed below.

- Coconut oil
- Olive oil
- Avocado oil

Snacks

The best snacks you can get come from nuts and seeds, such as pumpkin and sunflower seeds and mixed nuts. To make it more interesting, create your own trail mix pack. You can also snack on fruits and vegetables - for example, celery and carrots with hummus, or apples and cheese. As much as you can, make your snacks whole foods that contain healthy proteins and fats, along with beneficial fiber.

Top 5 Nutrition Tips

When thinking about nutrition, consider how well eating will fit into your schedule. Determining your time frame will help you eat the nutrients you need when you need them the most. Section out your meals using the suggested starches, proteins, fruits and vegetables, oils, and snacks, and determine the time of day you will work out. Below are more tips to get you through the day.

Eat Sufficient Protein Regularly

It is easy to believe that you need more protein than normal because you are building muscle, but that is not the case. In fact, you should be eating roughly the same percentage of protein in your diet that you would for carbs and fats. To find the best amount for you, eat 2 g for every pound of lean muscle. Ultimately, this means whether you weigh 150 or 200 pounds but have the same muscle mass, your protein intake would be the same.

You can find a rough estimate of your muscle mass by calculating your weight and height, using the percentage as the basis for the amount of fat in your body. From there, multiply that percentage by your weight to determine how much protein to eat. For a more professional and accurate percentage, contact your doctor. They can measure your muscle mass through an arm fat assessment.

Eat protein daily. Though many sources claim that you should mainly eat protein after or before a workout, when building muscle, your body requires a significant daily dosage of protein. Aim for 30% of your diet to consist of high quality protein.

Stay Hydrated

The amount of water you drink is highly dependent on your weight, height, and muscle mass. It is highly encouraged to drink as much as you can in a day, but be careful not to over drink, which can cause its own problems. The best way to determine how much water you should drink is to keep a journal and find which amount makes you feel the best. Remember that you lose a lot more water when working out, so add at least two cups of water for every hour you work out.

Build a Routine and Stick to It

One of the most difficult parts of maintaining a diet is boredom. After eating broccoli for three weeks, it can become tiresome, creating frustration. However, if you do not maintain a healthy routine, your muscle-building plan will fall apart. It takes at least three weeks for a new habit to form, so develop a sustainable schedule for at least a week to begin.

Find out your daily eating habits by keeping a journal without judgement. If you can accurately record how many calories you consume every day without pandering to the illusion that you can prevent yourself from eating too much, you can accurately determine where to fix your diet. Often, people eat little to nothing all day and pack on the calories at dinner. Though this approach works for some, it is often unmaintainable. Instead, find out what times of day you are hungry and develop a routine to refuel during those times. If you eat five times every day, consider reducing portions to fit into your diet routine.

Choose a diet schedule and caloric limit that is attainable. Many who want to lose fat quickly revert to the belief that they can seriously cut into their calorie intake to account for the change in diet focus. Not only does it become more difficult to deprive yourself of nutrients every consecutive day, but starving yourself also leaves your body more prone to sickness and unable to function at its highest capacity. Losing fat should not come at the sacrifice of your health.

Eat a Slight Calorie Surplus

You should be eating the same number of calories every day with slight variations on workout days. Your caloric intake, then, should become an average of what you consume on your off days and on workout days. On average, this is approximately a 200 - 300 calorie surplus. If you add cardio to your workouts, you can expect to increase that amount slightly to compensate for the extra work.

Consider Supplements

Though we have established that supplements are not generally necessary to build muscle, they can help the body if there is a deficiency in some macronutrients. You may also find that adding supplements to your diet will help you perform better. Consider adding a supplement to your diet to give you an edge, but do so with caution. Too much of any supplement can be damaging.

How to Build Muscle by Training

Though a proper diet is the place to start when building muscle, it is not enough. The only way to build muscle is through training. However, the wrong kind of training or using the wrong techniques can result in frustration when the body never changes. Many who fail to see gains after working for years are often aggravated and find it difficult to maintain a workout routine. It makes sense to feel angry when you are not reaching your goals. Here are the ways to gain muscle through training.

Progressive Overload

One of the most common mistakes in training is not increasing the difficulty of your weights over time. Those who stay at the same level for years often do not increase the weight size, volume, or frequency, preventing them from achieving change.

Muscles become accustomed to the same amount of weight when you use it for years. That is why you see people who lift 15 pounds perhaps developing tone but not increasing muscle size. Challenge your body to see what it can do. Likely, if you can easily lift 20 pounds, you can lift 25 pounds. Your muscles should feel tired after working out due to the extra strain. If you do not feel slightly sore from your workout yesterday, it might be time to up the weights.

Increasing the number of repetitions you perform will also help your muscles grow. You should complete approximately ten repetitions for every set you do. However, test your limits by seeing how many times you can repeat an action. If you can lift it more than 12 times, it is time to increase the weight. Remember, these repetitions must include proper technique. If you can lift a weight 15 times but your form starts to suffer after 10, maintain the same weight and aim for improved technique.

If neither of these muscle gaining techniques are working, increase the number of sets you perform. Generally, you should not exceed more than four sets. However, if you perform two sets, consider adding another set, increasing the continued strain on your muscles. While maintaining proper technique, try to work from a different angle. You may find that moving your legs further in a squat or holding your arm further from your body during bicep curls will work different muscles entirely.

As you become more accustomed to a regular training routine, increase the number of days you hit the gym. Your muscles still need time to heal, but the extra strain on the muscles will force them to adapt more quickly. Keep in mind that this is best used for a single problem area and is often used for a short period of time.

Mechanical Tension

Mechanical tension is the means by which muscles contract and expand. Using mechanical tension while working out is another way to improve your muscles, and it is often under appreciated. Consider standing up from a seated position. When you stand, your hip flexors and quadriceps contract, pulling you upward. Though your hamstrings do play a small part in pulling you to your feet, the majority of the work comes from the muscles knitting together.

One way to improve your workout through mechanical tension is by changing your range of motion. If, for example, you normally head for the bench press, consider changing it for a chest press using dumbbells. Though you perform the same action, dumbbells allow your arms to sink further than a bar would, forcing your muscles to contract further. You may find that this range of motion is more difficult, so be prepared to lower your normal weight limit.

Passive tension allows your body to adjust the level of force you put on your muscles. According to Greg Smith, a personal trainer located in London, England, "Passive tension is created when a two-joint muscle is stretched at one joint while it is forced to contract at the other joint" (2020). Performed correctly, this exercise allows your body to contract muscles that are uncommonly used.

The easiest way to achieve maximum mechanical tension is to simply increase the weight resistance. Just like with progressive overload, when you add weights, you are putting strain on your muscles. The muscles are forced to contract with greater force, increasing tension. If you increase your load by five pounds every week, you will see the effects of both mechanical tension and progressive overload training.

Metabolic Stress

Metabolic stress is all about how long you can continue to work. So, if you feel like you are going to throw up from the number of sets you complete, you are working with metabolic stress. Muscle builders who use this strategy focus on building lactic acid in their muscles and maintaining a high level of exercise for long periods of time. An increase in weight load, repetitions, and sets all factor into the effectiveness of metabolic stress during muscular training. Shorter times between repetitions also plays a large role.

Swelling in the muscles is a sign of metabolic stress. The muscles receive less oxygen during extended time under stress, which signals the body to produce water to fill the muscles, causing the cells to expand. Performing repetitions until you have to stop often indicates you will become more sore from metabolic stress.

Remember that you should not devote your entire workout to metabolic stress. You will soon tire, and it will do little good for your body.

Instead, work to improve a certain muscle group. If you attempt to work out your entire body with metabolic stress, you would be at the gym for hours, if not days. Professional athletes focus on one group at a time because the muscles fatigue quickly. Imagine performing the same motion constantly and with increased weight. Your body cannot handle too much all at once, and pushing too far could lead to extensive muscle damage.

Muscle Damage

If you do not push yourself to your limits, you will not see the benefits of muscle gain. The phrase "no pain, no gain" is accurate, to an extent. If you do not feel pressure on your muscles, you are not doing anything to help them. Muscle damage breaks down small muscle fibers, requiring them to build again to become better, as we've discussed. So, that's where the "pain" comes in - when those fibers break down. The "gain" comes when they are re-knit and repaired.

This damage is necessary to gain muscle. After all, your muscles must undergo damage for them to repair. The microtears in the muscles force the body to build them again, but stronger. However, it is possible for tears to become too large, often resulting in pain and the inability to use your muscles until they heal correctly.

The Importance of Macronutrients

We've talked about the macronutrients - carbohydrates, proteins and fats. Proper consumption of the three will assure muscle gain and fat loss. But, it's always "easier said than done," when we say that you should consume a high percentage of carbohydrates, then proteins, then fats. So, I've put together this simple meal plan to give you an idea of how it will look for you.

Example Meal Plan

Though this meal plan will not go into specifics, it will give you an idea of how to organize your meals throughout the day. Make sure you keep a journal of your eating habits to find the best distribution of calories for you. This is based on a 2,500 calorie diet.

Sample Macronutrient Meal Plan			
Meals	Carbohydrates	Proteins	Fats
Breakfast	10% - 250 calories	10% - 250 calories	0% - 0 calories
Lunch	20% - 500 calories	10% - 250 calories	10% - 250 calories
Dinner	20% - 500 calories	10% - 250 calories	10% - 250

The plan is ultimately up to you, so determine which meals are most important for your energy and play to your strengths.

Shopping List

Most of the ingredients and foods in this list might already be in your cupboard, but it's wise to check the grocery store for some important muscle-building foods that will help you succeed at the gym, and in relation to your muscle building goals.

- Whey protein
- Creatine
- Iron supplements
- Zinc supplements
- Berries (strawberries, raspberries)
- Milk and cheese (grass-fed is best)
- Chicken, grass-fed beef
- Whole grains
- Leafy greens
- Fatty vegetables, etc. (avocadoes, nuts and seeds, olives)
- Tropical fruits (mangoes, bananas)

CHAPTER 7:

THE SIMPLE PLAN YOU NEED TO LOSE FAT FOREVER

Losing fat is difficult. Millions of people struggle with obesity because it is difficult to change routines and find a diet plan

that will work well with your lifestyle. Even those who build muscle often find it difficult to lose the fat they have under their newly evident muscles.

Many people blame their metabolisms or claim that their genes are the reasons for their failure to lose weight. While these do play a factor in fat loss, they are hardly the only reasons. How you organize your life has a lot to do with your eventual success, and it might surprise you to know that losing fat is easy if you follow some simple guidelines.

Why You Can't Lose Fat

Fat plagues those who strive to gain a healthy physique but cannot quite get the handle on maintaining a healthy diet. They believe that enough exercise will magically cure their excess fat reserves. But, especially from what we have already discussed in this book, you should know that the majority of successful weight loss starts with a healthy diet combined with proper exercise. These two pillars are essential to gaining the body you always wanted.

Underestimate Your Caloric Intake

Many people who struggle with losing fat are often not looking at the foods they are consuming. Processed foods and unhealthy coatings of fat and sugar plague today's society, adding an extra layer of fat around the belt. The ingredients in fast foods and at the grocery store are either too difficult to wade through, or they are highly ambiguous, making it difficult to separate your foods into macronutrients.

It should come as no surprise, then, that most people underestimate how many calories they consume. It is easy to believe that you are making the most out of your diet by eating the right things, but this is not always the case. Even eating the most nutritious meals do not help your fat gain if you are not eating them in the right amounts. A caloric deficit is necessary to lose any fat, regardless where it comes from.

Though you already know that fried, sugary, and fast foods are bad for you in the long run, you may not know how big an impact these foods have on your caloric intake. You may be surprised how unhealthy some of your favorite foods are. A simple donut may cost you 200 calories and will not fill you up at the same rate broccoli might. Fried chicken, though delicious and high in protein, is covered in fried batter, making it unhealthy.

If you want to lose fat, track how many calories you consume every day. Smartphone apps, such as MyFitnessPal, are excellent resources to give you an accurate view of your average caloric intake. Remember that you must eat enough throughout the day to keep you energized, so eating the right foods is essential. If you are retaining fat, there is an excellent chance that it is because you are eating too much. Any excess calories in a meal, whether they come from donuts, steak or broccoli, causes a spike in your insulin levels, which causes the body to store those extra calories as one thing and one thing only....fat. So the quality and quantity of your food intake matters.

Overestimate How Much You Burn

We all want to feel as though our workouts mean something. When you hit the pavement for a run, it is understandable to feel justified in wanting that extra bite of cheesecake. However, you are likely not burning as many calories as you think you are.

One of the largest exercise culprits is cardio. It is estimated that you burn around 100 calories for every mile you run or walk, which means that, if you run five miles in an hour, you are only burning 500 calories. You can eat that number of calories when you hit the nearest burger joint. The truth is that you will not burn enough calories performing cardio than gaining muscle through lifting weights.

You may wonder how an athlete remains skinny, even though they consume their body weight in food every day. If you train like an athlete, then you can eat whatever you want and not gain fat. That is because they spend many hours every week improving their bodies through exercise. They lose fat by expending the calories they burn on a daily basis.

Not Eating Enough Calories

If you can lose weight by creating a deficit in your caloric intake, it only makes sense that you should be able to lose weight significantly faster by reducing it by an even larger amount, right? Contrary to popular belief, reducing the number of calories you consume to the point of incredibly small portions will not help you lose fat. As you train, your body requires fewer calories since your body weight changes. If you start out your routine by eating 1000 calories every day, your body has nowhere to lose the fat, and it will horde it instead.

The body's metabolism shuts down in the absence of food, preventing you from losing weight. If you do not eat enough, the body prevents you from expending more energy by making you feel sluggish and unmotivated. The body does not want you to fail, only to survive. If you dip below 1200 calories, you might find that your metabolism becomes considerably slower.

When on a low-calorie diet, it is often difficult to maintain a deprived caloric intake. Your body becomes tired and overly hungry, reaching for nearly any food source. If you have been without food in the past, even for a few hours, you may feel like the next thing you see will be the ideal meal. Your body sees this as an opportunity to gain more nutrition, so it jumps at the chance to eat, often causing you to overeat. The guilt from overeating turns into depression, which also causes overeating. The vicious cycle continues indefinitely.

Eat Healthy, Too Often

There have been multiple studies that show it is not the type of food you put into your body, only the caloric intake. One man lost 37 pounds eating Big Macs three times a week in three months, while another man lost 27 pounds over the course of ten weeks by eating mostly Twinkies (Strong Lifts, 2018). Many people, however, waste their time spending too much time eating healthy foods and not focusing on a caloric deficit.

The next time you go into a restaurant, look at the ingredients in the salad. Though the leafy greens are beneficial to the body, most restaurants make the salads unhealthy by adding croutons, rich dressings, and other additives. In the end, the salad is hardly healthier than anything else on the menu. Many people find eating healthy foods is much easier when adding an unhealthy spin, but the caloric intake becomes significantly higher than if you skipped the salad altogether.

As a disclaimer, it is important to eat healthy foods. You can only gain a healthy body by ingesting the right foods. However, many people take this to an extreme, negating the health benefits. Eat healthy foods whenever you can, but satisfy your hunger and palate by choosing comfort foods in smaller amounts. That way, you won't feel like you're in deprivation mode, and you're more likely to stick with the plan.

Eating Fewer Calories Than You Burn

The ultimate solution to losing fat is eating less. In theory, eating fewer calories than you burn is easy. The only requirement to eat fewer calories than you burn is to keep track of them, but it can feel difficult when you are not used to maintaining a calorie deficit. The key to keeping up with a calorie deficit plan is to hold out and hold on. As long as you can follow the necessary guidelines to eat fewer calories than you burn, you will lose fat in no time.

Track Your Calorie Intake

One of the best ways to cut down on eating too many calories is to keep track of what you eat. All you need to do is download an honest app that will give you accurate results about how many calories each food has, along with the macronutrients (carbs, proteins, fats).

Most of what you eat are the same things, which makes it easier to track how many calories you consume. If you love to eat pasta, section your consumption into smaller portions, allowing you to eat the same amount of food but over a larger period of time. The routine you develop from tracking the foods you eat most often will also make it easier to determine how much you should eat when you eat out.

The majority of your results are determined by what you do when you are not thinking. That is why it is easy to overeat. When you sit on the couch and enjoy one of your favorite movies or go out to the bar with some of your friends, you rarely think of how many calories you are consuming. Once you are aware of what you are eating, it is more difficult to cheat on your diet. So, even when you do not want to know your caloric intake and enjoy your time on the town, remind yourself to keep track of what you are eating.

Estimate the Number of Calories You Burn

The first step to estimating the number of calories you burn is to determine your basal metabolic rate (BMR). This will tell you how many calories you use while sedentary. Generally, people use around 1,500 calories from their daily life, which includes walking at least 2,000 steps every day. However, this number is highly dependent on age, sex, weight, and height. Many doctors and online sources can give you a rough estimate of the calories you burn doing virtually nothing.

Remember that most people lead sedentary lives. This is because office jobs do not require most people to move around enough, keeping them from walking around and burning calories. Adding weight lifting to your regimen does not burn a significant number of calories to bring you out of the sedentary lifestyle. That is where adding steps to your daily routine comes in, even if that means walking an additional 5,000 steps every day.

Once you have started eating less and more consciously, start to record the number of calories you burn when you work out. This is often a relief, letting you know that you are losing enough calories to make eating that extra dessert worth it. However, underestimate how many calories you actually burn. The calorie deficit from overworking when you worked harder than you estimated will give you an extra few calories you do not have to work off in the future.

Create a Caloric Deficit

The ultimate goal to lose fat is to eat less food than you burn. Determine the best number of calories to burn every day by following a simple rule: do not eat too much or too little. The table in Chapter 1 gives an estimated number of calories to consume daily, so use that as a rough estimator. You should never eat less than 1,200 calories for any reason. Starving yourself does not equate to health.

Stop Wasting Time on Cardio

Cardio is a blessing and a curse. It burns a moderate number of calories, but it usually takes a lot of time to burn those calories. Most people do not even reach a high level of effort since most gyms today have TVs and books and magazines to read when you work out. It is difficult to reach your top gear when you are distracted by something else. For the most part, if you do not have the time of day to put forth at least an hour of cardio, there are other things you could be doing with your time that are more effective.

Assuming you are training for a marathon, you will likely have burned enough calories to justify eating anything you want. However, regular people usually do not have the means to complete high levels of cardio. Do not feel as though you need to sacrifice your job to lose weight. Just skip the cardio and aim for weight lifting and calorie reduction.

Lift Weights to Retain Muscle

While it is important to lose fat, you do not want to completely eradicate your muscle with it. After all, you are likely to feel more attractive and healthy when you have some muscle to show for your efforts. So, when you go to the gym, hit the weights, even if it is just for an hour.

Cardio is a common resource for people who want to lose fat, but it does not build muscle effectively. It is also often boring, and you should not have to stick to a workout routine that you hate. Instead, use body weight and HIIT exercises to gain muscle while eating fewer calories. This will increase your metabolism and allow you to burn calories even after you finish a workout.

Frequently Asked Questions

Many people ask questions regarding their weight or style of working out and which exercise is most effective to help them reach their goals. As a personal trainer, I am often asked these questions regarding gaining muscle and losing fat. Here are a few of the most common questions and their answers.

How Does Slow Metabolism Hinder Me from Losing Fat?

The first step is to determine if you do, in fact, have a slow metabolism. Many people use this as an excuse when weight loss is difficult, but that does not mean it is always the case. Metabolism refers to the rate at which your body turns the nutrients in your body to energy. If you have a slow metabolism, your body cannot convert energy quickly, often turning excess nutrients into fat. You can tell if you have a slow metabolism by looking at your body. If you have difficulty building muscle (which means that you have spent many months trying to achieve muscle mass), you may have a slow metabolism. Typically, short, low-muscled people fall under this category.

The best way to increase your metabolism is to work out. When you lose fat and gain muscle, you are increasing the efficiency of your metabolism. This can be extremely frustrating for people who have struggled to lose weight for a long time, but if you keep at it, you will see results. Some people note that they do not see variable results until over a month has passed.

The routine is the same for people who suffer from slow metabolism and those who are blessed with high metabolism. The key is to create a caloric deficit and keep to it. This also means increasing the quality of your diet. The more foods you consume that will bring you more energy that you can use quickly when working out, the more likely it is for your metabolism to increase significantly. Consistency is key to keep your body from slipping back into a fat-storing factory. Lift weights and perform light cardio to get even more bang for your buck.

What Should I Eat to Lose Fat?

There are no magic foods that allow you to lose fat, otherwise there would be a booming industry and no one would be overweight. The secret, again, comes down to your caloric deficits. If you reduce the number of calories you consume, you will see your fat levels lower.

However, there are some foods that aid in losing weight based on their nutritional value. Whole grains are complex carbohydrates, which means that they pack a punch in the nutrient department and make you feel full after you eat them. Do not substitute whole grains for their processed counterparts like white bread or sugary cereals. Nuts are also commonly used as fat-fighting agents. They do not have many calories, but they contain large amounts of protein and fats, so will fill you up and give you energy. Lentils, lean meats, and dairy products also aid in reducing fat as they contain healthy fats and proteins.

Getting the most out of these foods comes down to how much you exercise. Though they can help you get the nutrients needed for the day, they are ultimately best suited for aiding your fat loss while working out. These foods will give you the energy to perform better.

Does Eating Fat Mean I Will Gain Fat?

A common myth states that you gain fat from eating the wrong kinds of fat, which are harmful to your body. In reality, fats are important to a healthy diet and eating them will not make you fat, unless you eat too many. Fats make you feel full at approximately the same number of calories as proteins and carbs, making them essential in maintaining weight loss. Keep your fat consumption low, but do not sacrifice it entirely for more protein and carbs.

Fat is created by excess nutrients in a system. When carbs, protein, or fats are introduced to the diet but are not properly converted to energy, your body saves them for another time. Therefore, it is vitally important to use the energy you put into your body.

How Many Times a Day Should I Eat to Lose Fat?

Your body uses a certain number of calories to chew and digest food. On average, you burn one calorie for every minute you spend chewing and an additional 10% of your overall caloric intake digesting the food. So, if you are eating a 500 calorie meal in 10 minutes, you are effectively burning 60 calories. Considering the number of calories you consumed, it hardly seems logical to say that eating multiple times every day has a significant impact on how much you ultimately burn eating and digesting food.

The key to losing fat is to eat as many times each day that it takes you to feel full without overeating. That could mean that you take three large meals or split them into five smaller meals. In the end, the quality of the food you consume will help you resist temptation to overeat. Sugary treats are common culprits for ruining diets as they have empty calories and do not fill you up. Stick to proteins, carbs, and healthy fats when you split your meals.

Another common myth states that you will gain more weight if you eat closer to bedtime. However, your body does not stop working when you hit the sack. Your metabolism continues to work throughout the night, making the time you eat less important. Studies have suggested, though, that you are more likely to consume extra calories when you eat closer to bedtime, so keep track to prevent weight gain.

How Do I Stop Snacking?

One of the best ways to stop eating junk food is to stop buying it. If you consider how much money you spend on junk food, the numbers might just convince you to stop. The next time you go out for a snack, think about what percentage of your paycheck is going into buying you a moment of pleasure. Putting it in terms of money is often a great motivator.

When you drink water more often, you are less likely to feel cravings. Most of the time, when you feel hungry, you are actually thirsty. Do not put your health on the line by only purchasing sports drinks, however. They often have large stores of sugar and deprive you of eating higher quality calories later.

Identify your triggers. Some people find that when they go out with friends, they are more likely to snack. This should in no way affect your social life, but being aware of what makes you eat more helps you reduce the number of calories you consume. If you find yourself returning to the same snacking traps, put some distance between yourself and your triggers. If you often get up for a midnight snack, place a temporary lock on your refrigerator that makes the effort inconvenient. If you snack when stressed, find a healthy outlet (like muscle building) that will put literal distance between yourself and junk food.

Binge eating due to excessive hunger is another reason many turn to junk food. The body starts to experience discomfort when hungry, which is a strong motivator for eating. Instead of battling through hunger and whittling away at your will power, eat only when you are hungry. Keep healthy snacks around to satisfy hunger pangs without compromising your diet.

When your body does not get enough sleep, it causes the brain to think irrationally. Your brain needs sleep to function effectively, and when it does not get enough, it turns to other methods to gain pleasure, including snacking. Getting little sleep also prevents your brain from making clear decisions. It becomes significantly harder to maintain willpower because your mind justifies small decisions that hurt your diet, like you need that extra coffee or you cannot attend the gym because you are too tired. Get at least seven hours of sleep every night to aid in weight loss.

Should I Weigh Myself Daily?

The decision is highly dependent on what you are trying to achieve. For example, if you want to lose weight, you should weigh yourself daily to make sure you are making progress. However, if you aim to gain muscle, you may see little changes on the scale from day to day. The short answer to the question is, you can if you want to.

Weight fluctuates daily. You may find that your weight moves up and down the scales significantly, even in a 24-hour period. Eating too much salt the day before hitting the scale may result in a higher weight. Also, dehydration and constipation are common reasons for weight fluctuations. So, you should not be using the scale as a measure of how much you are losing daily but as a tool to track your progress. Look at how things are moving on a weekly basis, versus emphasizing day-to-day fluctuations.

Do I Need to Count Calories to Lose Weight?

It can be frustrating when you count calories and realize that you have to take a lot of your favorite foods out of your diet. So, the short answer is no. There are many people who get along fine without counting calories and still lose fat. However, they follow the same principles that are outlined above: eat less and move more.

The reason for counting calories is to create a calorie deficit in your diet. If you can create a deficit in your diet without counting calories, you will receive the same results. However, before you stop counting calories full-time, look at how many calories there are in some of your favorite foods. You can more accurately underestimate calorie consumption with a more accurate understanding of foods' caloric value.

CHAPTER 8:

MAINTAINING MUSCLE MASS SO YOU DON'T LOSE IT, EVEN OVER 50

Losing muscle is a scary concept, especially for those who have seen how deteriorating muscles have affected loved ones. People over the age of 50 are more prone to muscle loss. But, it does not have to be your lot in life to lose muscle if you go through the proper training and keep up good habits.

Preventing Muscle Loss

The best way to maintain muscle mass is to go to the gym, but that is often easier said than done. There are so many excuses that seem logical at the time but eventually eat at your resolve to maintain a healthy level of muscle during your life. Remember, though, that you are responsible for the happiness in your own life. To prevent the deterioration of mind and body, resolve to prevent muscle mass today.

The key to maintaining muscle is to train at nearly the same levels you have in the past, but take a break every once in a while. Changing your routine may seem hard at first, but it is the first step to continuing a healthy lifestyle. The majority of the hard work is already behind you, so take advantage of the gains you have made.

Weight Training for Life

If you are new to weight training, check with your doctor before starting a new routine, especially if you have an injury. Starting weight loss over the age of 50 comes with its own struggles, including loss of muscle from a sedentary life and restricted range of motion. However, that should not stop you from starting your journey. Visit a physical therapist if you continue to struggle.

Most sources agree that you should work out two to three times per week, allowing enough time for your muscles to heal properly in between workout sessions. You can use whatever source is most comfortable to you since weight training is not restricted to lifting weights. If you are more comfortable using elastic bands or body weight, do what makes your body most comfortable.

Weight training is the only type of exercise that prevents the reduction of muscle mass over time. Aerobic exercise is a common go-to for many who are new to exercising because it gets your heart rate up and helps reduce weight. However, if you want to maintain muscle mass as you age, choose weight training over aerobic exercise. The best results, of course, come from incorporating a combination of the two exercises, giving you both brain and body health.

Focusing on weight training will also prevent you from getting injured. For instance, one of the most common causes of injury is falling. Since muscle training stabilizes your muscles, you will be better able to maintain a steady balance as you work out. Focus on muscles in the core, arms, and legs to increase flexibility in your body. Once you have established a healthy weight training routine, start to add aerobic exercise three to four times each week for significant health improvement.

When weight training, focus on how your body feels. If you feel pressure turn to pain, stop lifting weights immediately. As the body ages, tissues are not as sturdy as they once were, making muscle damage more difficult for the body to repair. You want to push your body to achieve impressive results, but it should not be at the expense of your health.

Get Enough Protein

As a weight lifter, it is important to get enough protein into your diet to account for your muscle gains. However, as you get older, ingesting enough protein is vital. The body needs the extra nutrients to build muscle and perform daily functions. It is estimated that older people need as much as 0.2 g more protein per pound than their younger counterparts.

Studies have shown that adults over 50 who consumed protein as 30% of their diet were better able to function as they reached ages of 70 and onward. They were less likely to have serious injuries, and they were better able to move around. The people who ate more protein in their diets also showed better health overall. Protein helps reduce the effects of aging.

A study conducted by Nuno Mendonca et al. (2008) discovered that increasing protein in aging adults even after a low to mild intake previously significantly improved their abilities to move and live alone. These individuals were also more likely to participate in activities such as walking, running, or hiking because they felt an increase in energy.

When maintaining weight, it is not as important to eat protein as before, but your muscles still need fuel for repair. Instead of consuming protein shakes, move to lean meats like chicken or fish. Replace protein supplements with lentils and beans. Unused protein shifts to fat if not used soon after consumption, so add only enough protein to your diet to maintain your level of fitness.

Eat Right

The better you eat as you age, the more likely you are to maintain muscle and perform daily activities without troubles. Aim for eating foods that will give you energy. After all, these are the foods that will keep you going when you are at the gym. You are less able to metabolize nutrient-lacking food as you get older, making weight gain more common. Find the foods you like best from every category (starches, proteins, fruits, vegetables, and fats), and increase your intake.

Keep track of how many calories you burn on an average day. Your basal metabolic rate is not equal to anyone else's, which means that, to create a wholly personal diet, you must calculate how many calories you burn doing nothing. Include an average amount of exercise you complete every day. If you increase your physical output, you must likewise increase your input.

Though it is not vital to weigh yourself every day, keeping track of your weight can help you discover how much you need to lose and which foods work best given the amount of weight lost. If you are careful with your caloric intake, you can still lose or maintain weight while sneaking a slice of pie into your routine. If you are over 50, however, remember to decrease the total amount of fat you consume daily.

Train Right

When starting out, many people fall into the trap of working out incorrectly. Though you may see some gains from this method, it is far more likely that you will neither gain as much muscle nor lose as many calories when you perform moves incorrectly. Thankfully, modern technology has made it possible for everyone to learn how to do any workout move recorded through video. Visit YouTube to discover how to move correctly to both help you gain muscle and prevent injury.

Another solution is to hire a personal trainer. Most gyms offer a personal training program that will give you the right exercises for your body type while helping you as you work out. The advantages of personal trainers cannot be understated. They know how each movement affects the way your body moves, and they help you feel better as you work out. They will also give you tips for gaining muscle for your body type, age, and sex, all invaluable information.

Even if you have been training for years, put yourself in front of a mirror to see how well you perform every technique. Seeing yourself do every exercise will help you improve and prevent injury. For example, squats are an excellent form of exercise that use body weight to create resistance when you bend your knees, working your legs. However, many bend their knees over their toes, which can be dangerous, often resulting in knee damage. If you watch your form in the mirror, you can see how far you must squat and how closely your knees are to your toes.

Be mindful of your body and its limits while exercising. If you feel hungry or thirsty before heading to the gym, eat a small snack and drink at least two glasses of water before performing any exercises. Not only is it difficult to maintain your usual pace when your body is not fully nourished, but you may experience light headedness and cramps as well. If you feel faint while working out, stop immediately and grab a glass of water. Next time you head to the gym, be sure to eat at least four hours before exercising.

You should be replacing the electrolytes and fluids in your body as you work out. Depending on the intensity of the exercise, you may sweat a considerable amount, and your body needs water to replace what was lost. Build up to longer exercise times over the course of a few weeks or months. Your body will become more accustomed to the exercise gradually, and there is less possibility for injury. You will also learn how much food you need to eat before working out to feel energized the whole time.

Get Enough Rest

Sleep is one of the most sought-after commodities in this fast-paced world. It is common to feel tired all the time if you are not getting enough sleep every night. So, imagine how much more detrimental the effect of little sleep has on your body if you are building muscle.

When you sleep, your body repairs the damage made to the body during weight training. The insulin-like growth factor hormone becomes active when you sleep, helping muscles repair and breaking down carbs to give you energy for tomorrow.

Achieving rapid eye movement (REM) sleep should be one of your most important goals. When your body shuts down, it enters a deep sleep, paralyzing your body. This is also the time when humans experience dreams. If you do not remember having dreams, it does not mean that you are not getting enough sleep. You may simply not remember them. But, you cannot achieve this intense level of sleep without long periods of rest.

When you begin training, you may feel like you want to stay in bed longer. Your body is telling you that it wants that extra hour to repair itself. Factor in at least nine hours of sleep every night to give your body time to prepare for the next day. If you are training for a marathon, you may notice that you require even more sleep. It is not uncommon for professional runners to spend 12 hours per day in bed.

The quality of your sleep also determines how well you will build muscle. If you have a highly irregular sleeping pattern (going to sleep at 9 PM on Wednesday then staying out until midnight on Friday), you will not receive all the benefits that come from a regular sleeping schedule. The body loves routine, and breaking routine will often result in difficulty sleeping. Though changing the time you go to sleep occasionally will not have a significant effect on your quality of sleep, consistently changing when you hit the sack will prevent proper muscle growth.

Limit Alcohol

Alcohol is another culprit that prevents proper sleep, ultimately leading to fewer gains (except when it comes to fat gains). Drinking a glass of wine a couple times per week will not upset your schedule much, but drinking every night will prevent you from achieving a good night's rest. Consider the last time you drank too much. Feeling hungover is a good sign that your body did not get the time it needed for repair.

Alcohol may result in muscle loss, if you are not careful. Alcohol prevents the body from producing hormones like estrogen and testosterone, which may hinder the growth of muscle.

Physique Maintenance

After you have gained muscle, it may feel like a step back to consider maintenance of that muscle, but that does not mean that you have to stop progressing. In fact, you should keep moving to see how far you can go. One of the greatest joys in life is achieving goals, and once you gain muscle, you can keep gaining muscle until you feel and look your best.

If you are unsure of where to turn next after achieving your muscle mass goal, focus on the enjoyment of working out. Once you start to exercise, it is difficult to stop without feeling repercussions in the body. Find new ways to exercise that will make you feel better and work harder. Attend local fitness classes or become part of a group that will encourage you to exercise and give you a push when you feel ready.

Remember, muscle maintenance does not mean giving up entirely. You may still find it useful to add weight when you train, but slow down the rate of change considerably. You will also not lose muscle if you choose to take a day or two off. Your body still works at a higher metabolic rate even after taking a week off, but do not make a habit of skipping weeks.

Nutrition

During the difficult stage of building muscle, your body constantly craves food, and intense workouts often give you the excuse to eat more. But what happens when you want to stop gaining muscle? Your caloric intake should level off, and you should be neither eating too much or too little. Use the BMR you determined in the first few chapters and stay at that steady pace. If you want a more general idea of how many calories to consume, follow the table in Chapter 1.

Once you have finished pushing your body to its limits, you can start eating the foods you want again. Remember, of course, that eating the right foods and exercising consistently are the most important ways to maintain muscle, but you are no longer trying to produce massive gains. Your body does not need as much protein to maintain muscle mass. Carbohydrates are not as necessary in your diet. Find a routine that works for you and be consistent.

Training

Training in muscle maintenance is also less structured than when training to gain muscle. So, if you had worked out four or five times each week, you can drop that number to three times, focusing on the whole body instead of individual muscles for every day at the gym.

Also, aim for higher repetitions. When you reduce the weight lifted and increase the number of repetitions, your body becomes more toned. This does not mean that you have to increase the overall volume of your workout. Stay within a limited number of sets and repetitions to keep the muscle you have and feel good. Complete no more than three sets at 12 to 15 repetitions, and focus on how your body reacts to the changes in pace. Most of the time, you will notice your body easily acclimating to the change in pace, and you might be surprised at your own strength.

Consider adding cardio to your workouts. Once you reach your muscle limit, cardio will still give you a good workout without forcing your muscles to grow further. Also, adding cardio to your routine will help you increase your mood and fitness level, allowing you to gain more endurance over time. Try running or interval training to increase your heart rate while pushing your body to a new limit.

Supplements

Your wallet will finally thank you when you reach the muscle-maintenance level. Suddenly, you do not have to dip into your savings to buy protein powder, expensive pre-workout drinks, or muscle-building supplements like creatine. Instead, focus on keeping the supplements that give you the correct nutritional value. If you only consume a multivitamin and an iron supplement, you will stay at the same level of fitness while sustaining your diet specifications. Note: if you are a woman and no longer menstruate, often iron supplementation is not necessary. Check with your doctor.

MEDICAL DISCLAIMER:

You are not reading a book by a medical doctor, nutritionist, or registered dietitian. The opinions expressed in this book, including texts, images, and videos, are generalized. They are presented "as is" for informational purposes only without warranty or guarantee of any kind. Adolpho Publishing LLC ("we", "our") makes no representation and assumes no responsibility for the accuracy of information contained on or available through this book, and such information is subject to change without notice. We are not liable nor claim any responsibility for any emotional or physical problems that occur directly or indirectly from reading this book. We are of the ability and use of conversation as per articles 9 and 10.

You are encouraged to confirm information obtained from or through this book with other sources. Our content is not a substitute for qualified medical advice. The supplement summaries in this book may not include all the information pertinent to your use. Before starting a diet, taking new supplements, or beginning an exercise program, check with your doctor to clear any lifestyle changes. Only your doctor can determine what is right for you based on your medical history and prescriptions. Not us.

Never disregard or delay professional medical advice or treatment because of something you read in this book. In case of medical emergency, contact a doctor or call 911 immediately. Again, you are not receiving professional medical advice.

AFTERWORD

Newcomers to weight lifting often get discouraged when they hear how many rules they have to follow or how much of their time is spent at the gym. With today's fitness craze, there is a lot of information that gives a variety of answers that may or may not help you gain muscle, especially when you are over 50. Sometimes it seems like the best way to muddle through the conflicting reports is to have a personal trainer at your side, guiding you through gaining muscle.

This book was designed for just that. I want you to know how to gain muscle by understanding how your body functions when exercising. Your body is capable of handling almost any obstacle, and *Shredded Secrets: Build Muscle, Burn Fat: 7 Cutting-Edge Nutrition Secrets You Need Even if You are Over 50 - The Bodybuilding Diet Plan for Men and Women* tells you how to get there.

When you follow the rules in this book, you will transform your body into a body of which you have always dreamed. All it takes is discipline and positive action.

The purpose of eating is to give you energy. Your goal when building muscle is to use the macronutrients available to you and make them work for you. The number of calories you consume dictates how much energy your body can produce from transforming macronutrients like carbohydrates, proteins, and fats into ATP, the body's energy source.

Eating complex carbs will fill you without making you overeat. Protein is essential for building and repairing muscle, and eating protein for approximately 30% of your diet will help you reach that goal. It is also vitally important to consume as many vitamins and minerals as possible through daily food consumption. Foods that are rich in iron, magnesium, B12, and other vitamins and minerals will not only help you perform longer but feel better as well. But, one of the most important substances to consume is water. Without water, you will not be able to exercise at all and your body will shut down.

The science of muscle growth helps you develop a routine that will help you build muscle faster and maintain it for longer. Muscle tension, metabolic stress, and muscle damage all promote muscle growth, given the proper stimulation. However, increasing the load for any exercise could result in injury if you are not consistent with your techniques. Hormones, such as testosterone and insulin-like growth hormone, are responsible for stimulating satellite cells, forcing the body to produce energy and work harder. To utilize these hormones to their highest potential, however, you must allow your muscles to rest. Rest allows them to knit together effectively and prevents injury.

The most common way to significantly increase muscle growth is through unhealthy practices, such as taking steroids. By themselves, the body does not produce enough hormones to increase the size of your muscles by large leaps. There are other factors, however, that could either aid or hinder muscle growth. Age, genetics, and hormones naturally determine how much your muscles will grow, but factors such as nutrition and training experience are the factors you can and should control.

Develop a routine to better time your nutrition. When you eat the right macronutrients at the right time, you will experience increased energy and muscle growth. It is important to eat before exercising to keep you energized for your full workout. During exercise, however, all that is generally needed is water to refuel your body when you sweat and breathe it out. After an exercise, take protein to give your body a head start into repairing your muscles. When it comes to rest days, consume roughly the same number of calories you would on exercise days. Muscle repair requires bodily rest and nutrient refueling.

The way we lose fat comes down to what we breathe out of our bodies. 84% of fat lost is carbon dioxide, which is expended when breathing hard during difficult workouts. The most basic way to lose fat, therefore, is to eat less and move more. If you aim to lose fat before gaining muscle, you must significantly reduce the number of calories you consume and exercise with mainly cardio. When losing weight during and after muscle gain, keep your body fueled with enough nutrients to maintain muscle while creating a slight deficit to lose fat. Increasing your protein intake will aid in losing weight while keeping your muscles strong. After all, if you starve yourself during or after gaining muscle, your muscles will deteriorate with the fat.

Protein is conclusively one of the best macronutrients for muscle gain. Therefore, taking a protein supplement is often necessary to bulk up. Creatine and citrulline malate are other options that help your body repair muscle more quickly and give you more energy as you work out. Calcium, vitamin D, HMB, and zinc are some of the most important supplements to take while gaining muscle. Most people do not ingest enough of these vitamins and minerals, preventing them from achieving optimal health. Do not fall into this trap. While many athletes use performance enhancers and herbs, they often do not play large roles in increasing muscle. Echinacea and ginseng are some of the most popular herbs, but their results vary wildly, making them unpredictable.

When it comes to building muscle, the first step is to add the right things to your kitchen. All members of the food group--starches, protein, fruits, vegetables, fats, and snacks--have a place in your kitchen, but make sure you are buying the right products to help you gain muscle safely. Find a routine that will help you succeed by eating the foods you enjoy while reaping the benefits.

To lose fat forever, it is all about the number of calories you consume. It does not matter if you eat nothing but cake and cookies all day as long as the total calorie consumption is less than your daily goal. Of course, I don't recommend that - but, you see my point. Consuming healthy foods, in a caloric deficit, will ensure proper nutrition and fat loss. If you are trying to gain muscle, forget about cardio and stick to lifting weights. You will see more muscle gain and it does not take as long to complete. Part of gaining muscle involves maintaining muscle, so work all parts of your body during weekly training.

Finally, you can maintain muscle by sticking to the workouts you have performed in the past but slowing your pace. You do not need to consistently lift larger weights to make it to keep the muscle you have. Instead, eat right, train right, get enough sleep, get enough protein, and limit your alcohol intake.

This book promised to deliver your way to muscle-building success, and *Shredded Secrets: Build Muscle, Burn Fat: 7 Cutting-Edge Nutrition Secrets You Need Even if You are Over 50 - The Bodybuilding Diet Plan for Men and Women* contains all the secrets you will need for the rest of your life. If you remember nothing else, remember to stay hydrated and keep moving forward.

REFERENCES

Almeida, C. F., Fernandes, S. A., Ribeiro, A. F., Keith Okamoto, O., & Vainzof, M. (2016). Muscle satellite cells: Exploring the basic biology to rule them. Stem Cells International, 2016, 1–14. https://doi.org/10.1155/2016/1078686

Andrews, R. M. (2018, April 4). All about nutrient timing: Does when you eat really matter? Retrieved February 21, 2020, from https://www.precisionnutrition.com/all-about-nutrient-timing#presale2

Appendix 2. Estimated calorie needs per day, by age, sex, and physical activity level. (n.d.). Retrieved February 18, 2020, from https://health.gov/our-work/food-nutrition/2015-2020-dietary-guidelines/guidelines/appendix-2/#table-a2-1

Auyda, T. (2018, February 28). The top 11 nutrients your body needs to build muscle. Retrieved February 19, 2020, from https://daily-burn.com/life/health/top-nutrients-build-muscle/

Bachus, T., & Macdonald, E. (2017, April 19). Meal timing: What and when to eat for performance and recovery. Retrieved February 21, 2020, from https://www.acefitness.org/education-and-resources/professional/expert-articles/6390/meal-timing-what-and-when-to-eat-for-performance-and-recovery

Bare Performance Nutrition. (2018, May 30). 7 Proteins To Eat To

Build Mass And Gain Muscle. Retrieved February 25, 2020, from https://www.bareperformancenutrition.com/blogs/nutrition/7-proteins-to-eat-to-build-mass-and-gain-muscle

Baum, I. (2018, October 20). Here's exactly what to eat on your rest day. Retrieved from https://www.menshealth.com/nutrition/a23939057/rest-day-diet/

Berardi, H. (2019, January 28). The science of nutrient timing! Retrieved from https://www.bodybuilding.com/fun/berardi54.htm?irgwc=1&utm_source=impact&utm_medium=affiliate&utm_cam-paign=ev-gl-1583875201478-acq&utm_content=1234031&ut-m_term=591986&irclickid=X2G18Dw9qxyOTza07OwzdzZ-UknX8hU3NSnFWE0

Bjarnadottir, M. A. S. (2016, January 18). 11 ways to stop cravings for unhealthy foods and sugar. Retrieved from https://www.healthline.com/nutrition/11-ways-to-stop-food-cravings#section9

Boorstein, B. (2019, June 25). Metabolite training (metabolic stress). Retrieved from https://evolvedtrainingsystems.com/metabolite-training-metabolic-stress/

Canter, L. (2018, December 13). The right way to fuel up before workouts. Retrieved February 21, 2020, from https://www.medicinenet.com/script/main/art.asp?articlekey=217254

Cava, E., Yeat, N. C., & Mittendorfer, B. (2017). Preserving healthy muscle during weight loss. Advances in Nutrition: An International Review Journal, 8(3), 511–519. https://doi.org/10.3945/an.116.014506

Chernoff, R. (2004). Protein and older adults. Journal of the American

College of Nutrition, 23(sup6), 627S-630S.
https://doi.org/10.1080/07315724.2004.10719434

Cleveland Clinic. (2019, May 21). Why You Shouldn't Weigh Yourself Every Single Day. Retrieved from
https://health.clevelandclinic.org/why-you-shouldnt-weigh-yourself-every-single-day/

Crump, K. (2018, September 20). What are macronutrients and why are they so important in strength training? Retrieved from
https://mystraightfitness.com/what-are-macronutrients-and-why-are-they-so-important-in-strength-training/

Dalton, S. (2016, December 16). Increasing iron intake to improve athletic performance. Retrieved February 19, 2020, from
https://www.healthline.com/health/increasing-iron-intake-improve-athletic-performance#athletic-performance

de Freitas, M. C., Gerosa-Neto, J., Zanchi, N. E., Lira, F. S., & Rossi, F. E. (2017). Role of metabolic stress for enhancing muscle adaptations: Practical applications. World Journal of Methodology, 7(2), 46. https://doi.org/10.5662/wjm.v7.i2.46

Fetters, K. A. (2017, October 20). 5 muscle building nutrients that aren't protein. Retrieved February 24, 2020, from
https://health.usnews.com/wellness/fitness/articles/2017-10-20/5-muscle-building-nutrients-that-arent-protein

Finn, C. (2019, July 17). How much protein do you need to build muscle? Retrieved February 25, 2020, from
https://www.menshealth.com/uk/nutrition/a754243/how-much-protein-should-i-eat-to-build-muscle/

Frestedt, J. L., Zenk, J. L., Kuskowski, M. A., Ward, L. S., & Bastian, E. D. (2008). A whey-protein supplement increases fat loss and spares lean muscle in obese subjects: a randomized human clinical study. Nutrition & Metabolism, 5(1), 8. https://doi.org/10.1186/1743-7075-5-8

Goulet, C. (2019, July 15). Progressive overload: The concept you must know to grow! Retrieved February 25, 2020, from https://www.bodybuilding.com/content/progressive-overload-the-concept-you-must-know-to-grow.html

Graham, J. (2019, June 5). Why older adults should eat more protein (and not overdo protein shakes). Retrieved from https://khn.org/news/why-older-adults-should-eat-more-protein-and-not-overdo-protein-shakes/

Greatlist. (n.d.). Genetic impact on building muscle. Retrieved February 20, 2020, from https://www.livestrong.com/article/332806-is-the-ability-to-build-muscle-genetic/

Greatlist. (2015, September 14). Fast-twitch vs. slow-twitch muscles. Retrieved February 20, 2020, from https://www.active.com/fitness/articles/fast-twitch-vs-slow-twitch-muscles

How can one maintain their physique? (2019, January 23). Retrieved from https://www.bodybuilding.com/fun/topicoftheweek133.htm

Inside Edition. (2017, February 3). Meet the ripped guy who eats just one 4,000-calorie meal every day. Retrieved from https://www.insideedition.com/headlines/21448-meet-the-ripped-guy-who-eats-just-one-4000-calorie-meal-every-day

Laron, Z. (2001). Insulin-like growth factor 1 (IGF-1): A growth hormone. Molecular Pathology, 54(5), 311–316. https://doi.org/10.1136/mp.54.5.311

Lee, J. (2020, January 23). The ultimate muscle building meal plan.

Retrieved from https://www.musclefood.com/blog/the-ultimate-muscle-building-meal-plan/#top-5-nutrition-tips

Leyva, J. (2020, January 1). How Do Muscles Grow? The Science of Muscle Growth. Retrieved February 20, 2020, from https://www.builtlean.com/2013/09/17/muscles-grow/

Magee, E. M. (2008, December 5). Good Carbs, Bad Carbs: Why Carbohydrates Matter to You. Retrieved February 18, 2020, from https://www.webmd.com/food-recipes/features/carbohydrates#1

Mawer, R. M. (2017, May 29). How Creatine Helps You Gain Muscle and Strength. Retrieved February 24, 2020, from https://www.healthline.com/nutrition/creatine-for-muscle-and-strength

Medline Plus. (2019, May 13). Nutrition and athletic performance. Retrieved February 20, 2020, from https://medlineplus.gov/ency/article/002458.htm

Mendonça, N., Granic, A., Hill, T. R., Siervo, M., Mathers, J. C., Kingston, A., & Jagger, C. (2018). Protein intake and disability trajectories in very old adults: The Newcastle 85+ study. Journal of the American Geriatrics Society, 67(1), 50–56. https://doi.org/10.1111/jgs.15592

Men's Health. (2014, June 20). 11 carbs that should be in your diet. Retrieved February 25, 2020, from https://www.menshealth.com/uk/nutrition/a747978/11-carbs-that-should-be-in-your-diet/

Michaels, J. (2012, February 29). Are you eating enough? Retrieved from https://www.jillianmichaels.com/blog/food-and-nutrition/are-you-eating-enough

Morgan, A. (2020, March 9). How to set up your diet: #4 nutrient timing; Meal frequency, calorie; macro cycling. Retrieved from https://rippedbody.com/nutrient-timing/

Muscle and Strength. (n.d.). Calcium. Retrieved February 23, 2020, from https://www.muscleandstrength.com/supplements/ingredients/calcium.html

National Institute of Health. (2019, December 6). Calcium: Fact sheet for consumers. Retrieved Winter 2, 2020, from https://ods.od.nih.gov/factsheets/Calcium-Consumer/

National Institutes of Health. (n.d.). Dietary supplements for exercise and athletic performance: Fact sheet for health professionals.

Retrieved February 25, 2020, from https://ods.od.nih.gov/fact-sheets/ExerciseAndAthleticPerformance-HealthProfessional/

National Institutes of Health. (2019a, August 7). Vitamin D: Fact sheet for consumers. Retrieved Winter 2, 2020, from https://ods.od.nih.gov/factsheets/VitaminD-Consumer/

National Institutes of Health. (2019b, December 10). Zinc: Consumer. Retrieved February 24, 2020, from https://ods.od.nih.gov/fact-sheets/Zinc-Consumer/

Nordqvist, J. (2017, November 27). What are the benefits and risks of whey protein? Retrieved February 24, 2020, from https://www.medicalnewstoday.com/articles/263371#dangers

Novak, J. (2017, December 21). Here's how long to rest between workouts. Retrieved February 20, 2020, from https://www.self.com/story/rest-strength-workouts

Nuts.com. (n.d.). How changing your diet can help eliminate body fat. Retrieved February 26, 2020, from https://nuts.com/healthy-eating/burn-fat

Own Your Eating. (2018, October 4). Calorie intake on rest days vs training days: Own your eating. Retrieved February 21, 2020, from https://www.ownyoureating.com/blog/calorie-intake-rest-days-training-days/

Parise, G., Mihic, S., MacLennan, D., Yarasheski, K. E., & Tarnopolsky,

M. A. (2001). Effects of acute creatine monohydrate supplementation on leucine kinetics and mixed-muscle protein synthesis. Journal of Applied Physiology, 91(3), 1041–1047. https://doi.org/10.1152/jappl.2001.91.3.1041

Patel, K. (2019, November 6). HMB. Retrieved February 24, 2020, from https://examine.com/supplements/hmb/

Patel, K. (2020, February 5). Citrulline. Retrieved February 24, 2020, from https://examine.com/supplements/citrulline/

Paturel, A. (2014, July 7). Sleep more, weigh less. Retrieved from https://www.webmd.com/diet/sleep-and-weight-loss#1

Penney, S. (2014, March 14). Calcium: For strong bones, muscle function, and so much more! Retrieved February 19, 2020, from https://blog.nasm.org/nutrition/calcium-strong-bones-muscle-function-much

Quinn, E. (2019, October 12). Your guide to strength training over age 50. Retrieved from https://www.verywellfit.com/strength-training-over-age-50-3119344

Robertson, J. (2018, February 23). Muscle: Magnesium Builds Muscle Mass. Retrieved February 19, 2020, from https://fitnessvolt.com/21207/muscle-magnesium-builds-muscle-mass/

Rogers, P. (2019, December 3). How to build muscle with bodybuilding hormones. Retrieved February 20, 2020, from https://www.verywellfit.com/build-muscle-by-manipulating-hormones-3498515

Rogers, P. (2020, February 12). Maintaining your muscle mass so you don't lose it. Retrieved from https://www.verywellfit.com/ways-to-lose-muscle-and-how-to-prevent-it-3498618

Ross, M. (n.d.). Genetic impact on building muscle. Retrieved February 20, 2020, from https://www.livestrong.com/article/332806-is-the-ability-to-build-muscle-genetic/

Russell, L. (2020, January 27). Fueling a Rest Day. Retrieved February 21, 2020, from https://www.hungryforresults.com/all-blog/rest-day-nutrition

Ryan, M. (2019, August 25). If You Have a Slow Metabolism, Here Are 5 Doctor-Approved Ways to Burn Belly Fat. Retrieved from https://www.msn.com/en-za/health/strength/if-you-have-a-slow-metabolism-here-are-5-doctor-approved-ways-to-burn-belly-fat/ar-AAGlBvD

Satrazemis, R. E. D. (2019, January 18). How Many Times Should You Eat a Day to Lose Weight? Retrieved from https://www.trifectanutrition.com/blog/how-many-times-should-you-eat-a-day-to-lose-weight

Scott, J. R. (2019, July 17). Calorie definition and why we count them. Retrieved February 18, 2020, from https://www.verywellfit.com/what-is-a-calorie-and-why-should-i-care-3496238

Senchina, D. (2018, August 31). Athletics and herbal supplements. Retrieved February 25, 2020, from https://www.americanscientist.org/article/athletics-and-herbal-supplements

Shapiro, J. (n.d.-a). Building muscle: How to start. Retrieved February 24, 2020, from https://www.julian.com/guide/muscle/workout-supplements

Shapiro, J. (n.d.-b). How to lose weight while maintaining muscle. Retrieved February 22, 2020, from https://www.julian.com/guide/muscle/weight-loss

Shapiro, J. (n.d.-c). The science of how to build muscle: Full guide. Retrieved February 20, 2020, from https://www.julian.com/guide/muscle/intro

Skerrett, P. J., & Willett, W. C. (2010). Essentials of healthy eating: A guide. Journal of Midwifery & Women's Health, 55(6), 492–501. https://doi.org/10.1016/j.jmwh.2010.06.019

Smith, C. (2019, April 8). The most nutritious fruits and vegetables. Retrieved February 25, 2020, from https://www.bodybuilding.com/fun/the-most-nutritious-fruits-and-vegetables.html

Smith, G. (2020, January 20). 3 Strategies for Optimizing Mechanical Tension. Retrieved from https://breakingmuscle.com/fitness/3-strategies-for-optimizing-mechanical-tension

Strong Lifts. (2018, December 3). How to lose fat quickly (12lb in 90 days). Retrieved from https://stronglifts.com/lose-fat/

TEDx Talks. (2013, October 11). The mathematics of weight loss | Ruben Meerman | TEDxQUT (edited version) [Video file]. Retrieved from https://www.youtube.com/watch?v=vuIlsN32WaE

The Mecca Gym. (2017, June 8). Bigger and stronger: The science behind muscle growth and strength. Retrieved February 20, 2020, from https://themeccagym.com/science-behind-muscle-growth-and-strength/

Tomboc, K. (2018, October 31). How dehydration affects your body composition. Retrieved February 18, 2020, from https://inbodyusa.com/blogs/inbodyblog/how-dehydration-affects-your-body-composition/

University of Wisconsin Hospitals and Clinics Authority. (n.d.). Eating for peak athletic performance. Retrieved February 20, 2020, from https://www.uwhealth.org/health-wellness/eating-for-peak-performance/45232

Valentine, M. (2019, September 19). 9 nutrients your body needs to get fit and build muscle. Retrieved February 20, 2020, from https://www.goalcast.com/2018/08/14/nutrients-body-needs-to-build-muscle/

Venuto, T. (2019, January 22). Training Or Nutrition: Which Is More Important? Retrieved February 18, 2020, from https://www.bodybuilding.com/fun/venuto4.htm

VPX Sports. (2019, September 4). Best fats for building muscle. Retrieved February 25, 2020, from https://bang-energy.com/blog/fats-for-building-muscle/

Weubben, J. (2019, November 11). The complete guide to pea protein powder. Retrieved February 24, 2020, from https://www.onnit.com/academy/pea-protein-powder/

Wuebben, J. (2019, November 11). The complete guide to rice protein powder. Retrieved February 24, 2020, from https://www.onnit.com/academy/the-complete-guide-to-rice-protein-powder/

Zaman, M. (2019, December 2). How sleeping can help you build muscle. Retrieved from https://www.shape.com/lifestyle/mind-and-body/how-sleep-affects-muscle-growth